Advance Praise for
Confessions of an Imperfect Caregiver

Confessions of an Imperfect Caregiver, perfectly encapsulates the *human* experience, not just the caregiver's. When we live in a world of worry, stress and self-doubt, where do we find the strength to go on? Bobbi's retelling of her caregiving years unfold in a beautiful answer to the questions posed by sickness, health, care, and loss.

Alexandra Axel, Media Director, The Caregiver Space

Written from the heart—not sparing the details, Bobbi Carducci presents the everyday challenges of being a loving caregiver. No topic is hidden or talked around. This is reality! By telling her story Bobbi has given us valuable insight into the confusing and often frustrating world of healthcare today. Read it for the story and use it as a guide should you be called upon to be "An Imperfect Caregiver."

Suzanne L. Walls, www.a-childs-book.com

...a testament to love, compassion, grace and courage in the face of often inconceivable challenges. ...Her tale is nothing short of heroic—invaluable for fellow caregivers. ...a must-read for anyone who has a family or has loved another person. A story for us all.

Erica Herd, Writer, Performer, Co-Author of the solo play, *Alzheimer's Blues*

Brutally honest and written from the heart, Carducci's intimate chronicle of caring for her father-in-law is a poignant story of strength, compassion, and humor that will linger with you long after you read the last page. Highly recommended for anyone caring for an elderly parent.

Jan Neuharth, author of the *Hunt C*

...opens the door so others can get a glimpse of what goes on behind closed caregiving doors. ...a testament to the power of hope, faith and love. They are the driving forces that enable Bobbi to continue on her caregiving path despite the ominous challenges. Like the millions of caregivers across the globe, she is, in my opinion, a most amazing - and perfectly human - imperfect caregiver!

Lynn Greenblatt, CaregivingCafe.com Information Resources Support Solutions

This book moved me from tears to laughter to compassion. This book is all about Rodger; this book is all about Bobbi; this book is all about Mike. Bobbi has somehow plaited these three lives into an amazing story of caregiving.

Sharon K. Garner, Copyeditor, Proofreader, and Author of *Pele's Tears, Sanctuary, River of Dreams, Lokelani Nights, The Spaniard's Cross*

This is a brutally honest portrayal of caring for someone with mental illness and dementia. An unpredictable roller coaster ride, Carducci describes her dramatic journey with love, humor and humility.

Donna Thomson, Author of *The Four Walls of My Freedom, Lessons I Learned from a Life of Caregiving.*

This story brought tears to my eyes so many times. Bobbi's words told of her genuine care and love for her father-in-law. I found myself identifying with her by thinking of my own struggles caring for my mother. Her words were honest but at the same time kind. I can't wait to share this book with my caregivers support group!

Bev Antwine, Family Caregiver

... remarkably courageous book.... I hope that whoever takes care of my final years will have read this book.

David Sackrider, Journalist

CONFESSIONS OF AN IMPERFECT CAREGIVER

BA Carducci

BOBBI CARDUCCI

To Florine —
One Caregiver
to Another —
Blessed Be

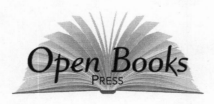

Open Books
PRESS

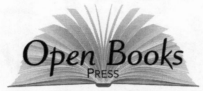

Published by Open Books Press, USA
www.openbookspress.com

An imprint of Pen & Publish, Inc.
Bloomington, Indiana
(812) 837-9226
info@PenandPublish.com

www.PenandPublish.com

ISBN: 978-0-9859367-7-8

This book is printed on acid free paper.

Printed in the USA

DEDICATION

To Rodger

"That in every hour you may be close to God.
This is my wish for you and those who are close to you.
This is my hope for you, now and forever."
From an old Irish blessing, author unknown.

P.S.: I hope that now it does make sense.

AUTHOR'S NOTE

This is a true story reconstructed from memory. I have changed the names of all medical personnel in this book to protect their privacy. These are my memories and may differ from their memories of the same conversation.

ACKNOWLEDGEMENTS

Although this is book is primarily about Rodger and me there is another person who was as much a part of it as we were. My wonderful husband, Rodgers dedicated son, Michael Carducci, supported us both in every way possible. He not only provided a loving home for his father, he became the caregiver's caregiver, often bearing a double burden when Rodger and I needed his strength and understanding at the same time.

Michael, you are my love, my light, and my inspiration. I am grateful every day that God gave me you.

❧

I wrote Confessions of an Imperfect Caregiver for the millions of caregivers and those who will become caregivers around the world facing the hardest job they will ever love.

Caregivers, if you learn anything from my story, I hope it's the understanding that you are only human and that sometimes being a little bit crazy is exactly what's needed in the moment.

❧

I could not have completed this book without the support and guidance of some very talented writers and mentors. I can't possibly list them all here, but if you are a member of Pennwriters or the Round Hill Writers Group, I mean you.

Special thanks go to Ramona DeFelice Long, Susan Meier and Lorraine Henderson all of whom believed in me and challenged me to get the work done. I am proud to have each of you as a friend and teacher.

Chapter 1

"Hey, give me my medicine. It's mine. Give it to me now!" my father-in-law called from the top of the stairs.

I groaned inside. *Not again. How many times do I have to tell him the same thing? Shut … up. Shut up. Shut … up. Dear God, please make him shut up.*

I reversed direction, and instead of reaching toward the shelf to put away a glass I'd removed from the dishwasher, I filled it with water and drank deeply, trying to drown the words before they could escape into the air.

Don't say it. Don't even think it. My face warmed from the rush of adrenaline coursing through me as I struggled to get my emotions under control. The deep, undeniable anger I was struggling with came out of nowhere, and I couldn't understand why it was surging through me now. We had been through hell the past several months, but all that was over and things were getting better.

This is so wrong. What's happening to me? The words "fight or flight" popped into my head. *What happens when you can do neither?* I wondered, sudden tears coursing down my face and sliding off my chin to mingle with drops of icy water I'd spilled on my pajama top.

"Do you hear me?" my father-in-law repeated, shuffling toward me, the *shush, swish, shush* of his worn slippers punctuating every word. Suddenly I hated that sound. "I can take my medicine by myself. It's too much trouble for you."

"I heard you," I answered.

I heard you this time and the last time and the time before that. I heard you yesterday and last night and at least ten times every day since you came home from the hospital. I hurried to dry my tears on my sleeve before he saw them.

Not that he'd notice, the mean little voice inside chided. *He lives in his own world and you exist only in relation to his needs. He doesn't even like you. You heard him talking to the nurses. You were useless.*

All you did was sit and stare at him all day. You fed him like a baby and nagged him all the time just like that other lady, the one who said, "Swallow, swallow, swallow, chew, chew, chew, and take small bites."

"I can't let you take your medicine on your own anymore, Rodger," I explained, just as I did every time he'd bring it up. "We let you do it before and you fooled us. You spit it out and got very sick. You almost died. I can't let you do that again."

"Yeah?"

"Yes. You were in the hospital for a long time."

"I remember. I had pneumonia." I didn't know if he actually remembered or not. His memory was so spotty and his determination to hide it so strong, it was impossible to tell what he recalled and what he pretended he knew.

"And before that you were on the psychiatric ward with the crazy people. Do you remember that part?"

"When I lived in Pittsburgh I went berserk one time."

"You went berserk here too, and that's why I give you your medicine now. I can't take a chance you'll get sick again." I handed him the small cup of applesauce containing his midmorning dose and watched carefully as he swallowed every bite.

"I know you don't trust me," he said, heading back upstairs to his room, "but think about it. I'm okay now and I can take my medicine by myself."

No you can't. And maybe I can't take care of you either. Why in the world did I ever think I could do this? I've made so many mistakes in my life. I failed at my first try at being a wife and made huge mistakes as a mother and a daughter. Hell, my own father chose a new family over a relationship with me and hasn't been heard from in years.

"God help us both," I whispered as the memories came flooding back.

"They both bitch at me all the time," Rodger had said, unaware I'd come back to the hospital to feed him dinner. "But she's the worst. She thinks I'm a baby. She's no damn good. I know all about women like her. No damn good. And look at the crap she brings. Flowers and cards and this damn thing."

Just then the little teddy bear I hoped would cheer him up sailed through the doorway of his hospital room.

Susie, his day nurse, came out a moment later and scooped it up. "He didn't mean that," she said, walking over and putting a hand on my shoulder.

"I know," I answered, surprised by the hurt his angry words had caused. "He's been through a lot in the last year."

"From what I read in his charts, you both have. He was up on the psychiatric floor for eight weeks then home for two days before coming back in with pneumonia. He spent a week in ICU and now he's here in step-down, still recuperating and undergoing more tests to find out if his swallowing problem was caused by a small stroke. I see you here every day. Your father is lucky to have you. Many of our patients have no one. Just remember you have to take care of yourself too."

"I will once we know he's going to be okay. And, for the record, he's my father-in-law. He came to live with my husband and me when my mother-in-law passed away last year. Caring for him is now my full-time job."

"Well, I say again, he's lucky to have you. God bless you and your husband—and don't let him fool you. He's glad you're here, even if he won't admit it."

Before I could comment either way, Susie was off to tend to her next patient.

I forced myself to smile, and swallowing my dismay over what I'd just heard, I went into the room he shared with three other disabled veterans.

"Hi, Rodger. How are you feeling today?"

Before he had a chance to answer, the man in the bed directly across from him spoke up. "Hey, welcome back." He grinned.

"Hello, Mr. Johnson. Are you still here? I thought you were going home today."

"I was supposed to but they say I need another day or two. I don't mind though. Looking at you makes me feel like I'm seventy again."

I chuckled at the left-handed compliment. "Thanks, I think. Let me know when you feel like you're fifty and we'll go dancing."

"It's a date," he promised, pretending to mark a day on an imaginary calendar.

I turned my attention to the other side of the room only to find that my father-in-law had drifted off to sleep. Or pretended he had. I decided that either way it was best to let him rest. I'd take advantage of the quiet and read until it was time to feed him again.

After going over the same two paragraphs four times, I gave up. The clicks and beeps of various monitors were too distracting. Instead, I let my gaze wander around the sparsely furnished hospital room. All four beds were in use. In addition to Mr. Johnson and Rodger, Joe Adams had the bed on the left by the window, and Pete Smith had the one across from him. Joe, a frail little man in his nineties, had a habit of taking out his IV whenever he had to go to the bathroom. As sick as he was, he refused to use a urinal or a bedpan, stating firmly that he was not an invalid and could manage to take a leak on his own, thank you very much. Each time he got up, he'd pause at the foot of Pete's bed, bow his head for a few seconds, then snap off a perfect salute to the now unconscious man lying there. Pete had never spoken or acknowledged Joe in any way. Pete's wife had been at his side constantly to offer a sip of water or adjust his pillows. Sadly, every day he'd taken another step back in his recovery. Now the only sign of life was the slight rise and fall of the thin blanket that covered him.

I tried to imagine these men as they'd been in their youth. They were the warriors, the brash young men who'd marched off to save the world when it needed it most. Between fierce battles they'd flirted and danced the Lindy with beautiful young women who'd promised to wait for their return. I sent a silent thank-you to each of them and said a prayer that they'd get a chance to go home again.

A ripple of movement from the direction of Rodger's bed drew my attention. Shock at what I was seeing sent a chill across the back of my neck and goose bumps racing down my arms. Still not quite awake, he'd begun to move. His head lifted off the pillow and started to weave side to side in a slow elliptical motion. Then his arms rose from his sides and his hands met above his head with the delicate grace of a figure skater preparing to go into a spin.

No. It can't be. It's my imagination. Everybody moves in their sleep, I thought.

But even as I tried to convince myself that what I feared wasn't happening, the movements increased in speed and intensity—and I knew he was off his medication again.

I rushed out of the room to ask Susie how this could have happened, only to find out that there had been a shift change and Susie was gone for the day.

"Who sees to Mr. Carducci's care tonight?" I asked.

"I do," one of several unfamiliar nurses, busy reviewing charts, replied. "Is there a problem?"

"I think so. I was just in his room and there are signs he's not taking his Zyprexa. Are you crushing it and giving it to him in his food?"

"He's been getting all his prescribed medications and he's been very compliant. There's nothing in his chart to indicate he ever refuses to take it."

"He's supposed to get it in applesauce. If you don't give it to him that way he hides it in his cheek and spits it out when you're not looking. I'm telling you he's not taking it and that could be very dangerous. He just spent eight weeks in the psychiatric unit. When he was admitted, he was ranting and severely delusional. He was so far gone, the doctors were afraid we'd never get him back."

"I didn't know that."

"How could you not know? Isn't it in his chart? My God, he wasn't out of the psychiatric ward for more than two days before he was readmitted with pneumonia. It can't be that far back in his records."

"Let me check on this and I'll get right back to you. Are you his daughter?"

"No. I'm his daughter-in-law. He lives with my husband and me."

"In that case I don't think I can discuss this with you. There are issues of privacy we must abide by."

"Yes you can discuss this with me," I said, taking a deep breath in an attempt to remain calm. "My husband and I have a medical power of attorney that gives us authorization to speak on his behalf. I'm listed as the primary medical contact because I take care of him at home while my husband goes to work every day."

"You should provide the hospital with a copy of both of those documents so they can be inserted into his file."

"We did. They're in there."

"I'll check on that too. Just give me a few minutes to verify all this and I'll get back to you."

I turned and stalked back to the room. I didn't want to wait for answers, not again. I needed to know that when I left the hospital each night he'd be getting the care he required.

He was wide-awake when I got to his bedside, eyeing his dinner tray. "I can feed myself," he snapped.

"No. I'm sorry, you can't. The doctor wants me to feed you so you don't eat too fast. You can't swallow very well and he's worried you'll choke."

"They think I'm a baby. Chew, chew, chew, swallow, swallow, swallow. It don't make sense. I know how to eat."

To prove his point he grabbed the spoon off his tray and started shoveling mashed potatoes into his mouth as if he hadn't eaten in a month. Immediately, he coughed and wheezed, his eyes watered, and his face turned a deep shade of crimson.

"Open up," I said. Using my fingers as carefully as possible, I removed a big hunk of saliva-diluted potato from the back of his mouth, grabbed all the silverware off his tray, and went to the sink to wash my hands. "Are you ready to let me feed you now?"

"Do what you want. You're just like that lady. You think I'm a baby."

I wanted to reply that he was behaving like a baby but I bit my tongue, reminding myself that he was old and sick and more than a little bit crazy. A lifetime of schizophrenia had left him deeply suspicious of everyone, and things were getting worse as old age and a number of chronic illnesses began to cause him even more stress.

"I don't want no more," he said after eating less than half of what was on his plate. "I can't eat much."

"Try a little more. Please? You need food to get well."

"I said no."

Rather than push him, I set the tray to the side, intending to get him to eat more in a little while.

Just then another unfamiliar nurse came into the room. "Mr. Carducci, you have to eat if you want to get better."

"No you don't understand—" I began.

"And you," she interrupted, "can't let him get away with this. He has to eat. Watch this," she ordered. She mixed three pats of butter and two sugar packets into the mashed vegetables on the plate and set the tray in front of him. "He's not a baby. He can feed himself. He's being passive-aggressive because you're his daughter. The longer you enable him, the longer he stays here. You should know that this isn't a good place for him. Hospitals are full of germs and he's too weak to fight them off."

I was about to set her straight on the enabling comment when Rodger choked. This time his face turned blue, and he vomited the greasy, oversweet vegetables all over himself.

"I tried to tell you," I shrugged, feeling a little smug at the nurse's shocked expression. "He has a problem swallowing and he's not supposed to feed himself because he overfills his mouth and then he chokes. That's why I let him stop for a while."

"I didn't know—"she began.

this latest setback. I wondered how many pills he'd thrown away this time and how long it would take for the drug to take effect again.

The cool evening air felt good on my face as I walked to my car. It helped ease the tension that had turned the muscles across my shoulders into taut steel cables. I needed to get home, eat a decent meal, and take a long, hot shower before the twinge behind my right eye became a headache that would keep me awake all night. But, once I got to the car, instead of starting it and driving the thirty-eight miles to get there, I sat in the darkening parking lot trying to figure out who the man really was that I'd welcomed into my home with love and affection.

For fifteen years I'd known him as my gentle, henpecked father-in-law. A man who longed for a little peace and quiet and always seemed eager to please. As saddened as I was by my mother-in-law's passing, I had believed that living in my home, free from the constant yelling and criticism, he'd come out of his shell and begin to enjoy life.

The first time I met him, when Mike and I first started seeing one another, he reminded me so much of someone dear to me that I felt as if I'd already known him for a long time.

Mike was living with his parents then, renting a large room on the third floor of the row house he'd grown up in, while looking for an apartment closer to work. We'd spent the afternoon together, and then he'd taken me to his room to show me his drum set and to play a few songs before I had to go home to my kids. Recently divorced and not used to dating, I was shy and unsure of myself. I wasn't comfortable being there at all and was relieved when he played the last note and offered to walk me to my car.

Descending the stairs, I noticed just the toes of a man's shoes, cheap, black, and rubber-soled. Then white socks, sagging around his ankles, came into view. His pants were navy blue. Since he was still seated, I couldn't confirm that their seat was almost worn through, but I knew instinctively that would be the case. *It's just the same with the brown pair he wears when the blue ones are in the wash,* I thought.

I watched him dig his heels into the footrest of his chair, easing the back upright so he could stand and offer a hand in greeting. A too-large brown belt circled his waist, welts of strain scarring the surface at various places, marking recent fluctuations in his weight. His shirt was a whisper-thin old thing, tucked inexpertly into the baggy pants he pulled up to a height only very old men find comfortable.

I felt a smile of recognition cross my face when his features came into view. Everything about him reminded me of my Uncle Louie. The fact that Louie was not just my uncle but my great-uncle, my personal godfather, and the only Italian in my big Irish family made him appear to be a man of epic proportions. He was shorter, darker, fatter, and far more interesting than any of the skinny, red-headed, freckle-faced men who chased after us when my brothers, sister, and cousins and I couldn't contain our wild selves a minute longer and tried to uphold the age-old Celtic tradition of fighting like a bunch of hooligans.

Whenever I'd stay with my godparents for a weekend, Uncle Louie would let me sit on his lap while he drank a beer or a highball. He even let me have a sip now and then. I didn't like the taste of either one but I never told him so. I had an idea in my head that sipping whiskey just naturally went along with watching the Friday night fights, and I wasn't about to risk losing that privilege for anything.

While Uncle Louie's gaze remained glued to the tiny black-and-white TV screen, I'd watch the crinkly lines around his eyes deepen each time he'd take a drag off his Camel cigarette and wonder how he got those puffy little bags to grow beneath his lower lashes like that.

My God, I thought as Mike began the introductions, *even his chair looks the same.*

"Dad, I'd like you to meet Bobbi."

Shaking off the memory of one person in order to acknowledge the presence of another, I greeted the man who would become my father-in-law, convinced I'd seen something familiar in him. *They have the same light in their eyes,* I thought with affection.

Sitting in a hospital parking lot so many years later, I was just beginning to discover how very wrong I'd been.

Had he been pretending all these years? Is the real Rodger the one who announced to the nursing staff that I'm useless and no damned good? Does the medicine he takes every day allow him to be himself, or does it mask his true nature? Who is this man who lives in my house and paces the halls late at night?

As hard as I tried to block out the thoughts, I couldn't stop the images from coming. Flashes of movie maniacs appeared, unbidden. Norman Bates from *Psycho* leered through a curtain of memory only to be replaced by rapid-fire clips of Jack Torrance careening through the halls of the Overlook Hotel in *The Shining*.

"Stop being ridiculous," I said, shaking off the mood I'd created and starting the car.

As I turned onto the highway I told myself that my thoughts and the fact that I was now talking to myself in an otherwise empty car were more an indication of my mental state than his.

I knew from my research that schizophrenics aren't the knife-wielding lunatics often portrayed in movies. Most of them are timid, introverted people who want to be left alone. Unfortunately, very often when they get their wish they end up homeless, in the hospital, or in jail. And sometimes, even when they aren't left alone, those things happen.

Where did I go wrong? What did I miss and how can I make sure this doesn't happen again? Those questions and more went unanswered as I covered the miles between the hospital and home, my mind and body too tired to cope with the guilt I felt at that moment. Despite all my good intentions, I'd let him down.

"Just think about it," Rodger called out just before entering his sitting room. "It's too much for you to worry about. I can take my medicine myself."

Can you hear me, God? I prayed, turning my back on him and putting the rest of the dishes away. *Hold me in your love and light and take this anger away. And one more thing. Please, for just little while, can you make him be quiet?*

Chapter 2

The sound of a morning news program coming from Rodger's sitting room signaled that at least part of my prayer had been answered. If all went well, he'd alternate flipping through the channels on his TV and napping until it was time to come down for lunch. A quick glance at the clock told me I had almost three hours before he'd try to talk me into giving him control of his medicine again. In the meantime I had work to do. Monday was laundry day, and once I got that going it would be time to create some leftovers.

I paused for a moment and looked out one of the tall windows in the two-story family room adjoining the sunny kitchen. The view is always a treat but especially so in the early morning and at sunset. I could hardly believe I was looking at such a beautiful setting from inside my own home.

Mike and I had come a long way, surprising a lot of people who were convinced our marriage wouldn't last. And they'd had good reason to think as they did. When we met, I was a thirty-three-year-old divorced mother of four. He was twenty-four and happily single. No matchmaker in the world would ever have put us together. I believe we ended up together because it was meant to be.

Deciding to end my marriage to a man I'd married at seventeen had not been easy. But, after sixteen years of trying to make it work, I realized things were never going to change. He'd become a mean drunk, and when he was sober he was still an ill-tempered, suspicious man, quick to anger and impossible to please. I had to get out and, more importantly, I had to get my kids out. To this day I have moments of regret that it took as long as it did to take that giant leap into the unknown. Then I remind myself that based on how things have turned out, the timing was perfect.

"You better think twice about leaving me," he'd warned, eyeing me up and down with a look of contempt the night I told him it was over. "No man in his right mind is going to want you. Look at you. You're not young anymore. You never were much to look at, and now you've got all these kids. If you divorce me, you'll end up alone for the rest of your life."

I believed him. Before finding the courage to file for divorce I had to come to terms with the idea of being the single mother of two teenagers and two elementary school children. It would mean years of sacrifice and many long, lonely nights. It would be the hardest thing I'd ever done and I was terrified of what might lie ahead, but I also knew that whatever it was it would be better than what I lived with then.

"Good." I answered, squaring my shoulders and looking him in the eye. "If having a man in my life means living like this, I'd rather be alone. Now get out."

Surprised by my response, but apparently at a loss as to how to respond, he turned and headed for the door. I heard him muttering through the screened front window as he walked to his car.

"I'll be back. Once she finds out she's not so smart, I'll be back." The screech of tires as he pulled away from the house transformed his half-whispered words into an angry promise. Like most of his promises, nothing ever came of it.

Not long after the divorce was final, I arrived at the night deposit of the bank at the same time as a handsome man I'd often seen in the restaurant where I worked as a manager. We talked for a while and something clicked between us. He invited me to meet him for coffee and ice cream a few nights later. He didn't know it at the time, but that particular invitation was perfect for me. I love ice cream and never say no when it's offered. I was relieved he didn't suggest we go to a bar. I accepted his invitation and looked forward to spending some time away from the kids for a while.

We talked for a long time that night, or truth be told, he did. I listened and watched him nervously tie straw wrappers into knots. *He's nervous,* I realized when the first scrap of paper disintegrated in his hands and he reached for another straw.

I found the idea that a man like him was afraid of me very

amusing. He was powerfully built, and I knew from our brief talk the night we met that he studied karate and had won a number of trophies in competition. I'd just come out of a marriage where every word and gesture I made had been scrutinized for hidden meanings and signs of disrespect. I was the one who'd needed to be afraid. Sitting across from Mike in a family diner, eating ice cream while he tried to impress me, was the nicest thing that had happened in a very long time.

"What?" he asked, pausing midsentence.

"What do you mean?"

"You're smiling at me and you're blushing." He laughed. "What are you thinking?"

"I am not blushing," I insisted, despite the warmth spreading across my face and neck.

"Yes you are." He grinned, his smile making my heart beat a tiny bit faster. "Come on, tell me," he teased.

"I was wondering …" I stopped, afraid to admit what had been running through my mind.

"You were wondering…" he prompted. "Go on."

"I was wondering what it would feel like to kiss you." I blurted before I could stop myself.

Then, horrified that I'd actually said it out loud, I prayed the floor would open up and swallow me. When it didn't, I forced myself to look at him across the table, hoping that somehow he hadn't heard what I said.

"Well, now," he said, trying to hide his own blush behind a menu, "that's not what I was expecting you to say." His eyes sparkled with amusement as he put down the menu and called for the check.

"What were you expecting?" I asked, laughing along with him.

"I forget, but it doesn't matter anyway," he assured me, "because I like your idea better. Let's get out of here."

After that we couldn't deny the attraction between us, but we knew it wouldn't last. We managed to convince ourselves we'd be okay when it ended and decided to enjoy our growing friendship. We never dated in the traditional sense. Most of the time we spent together was in the company of one or all of my children. My youngest daughter, Kelly, was convinced he came to our home to see her. I didn't try to dissuade her. It helped us keep up the pretense of being just friends. Mike was great with all four of the children right from the beginning. He never talked down to them or tried to impose himself upon them in any way. He didn't have to. He liked them and they liked him. He'd get down on the floor and play race cars with my eight-year-old son, also named Mike, and let six-year-old Kelly tie a scarf on his head and giggle at how silly he looked. He'd bring tapes of his favorite music to share with fourteen-year-old Patrick, who was teaching himself to play the guitar. They connected through their shared love of music and appreciation for bands like Kiss and Black Sabbath—music that Mom wasn't supposed to like and didn't understand.

With sixteen-year-old Colleen, he was like an indulgent big brother. Teasing one minute and protective the next. She's the only one who got her father's coloring. Her brothers and younger sister are all blue eyed and fair, with varying shades of blonde and red in their hair, like my family. So, with her dark hair and slightly olive-toned skin, she could have passed for Mike's little sister. I loved to hear their easy banter and watch him help her with her homework.

One afternoon after we'd had been seeing each other for more than a year, we were all in the living room playing a board game when I realized everyone was laughing out loud, including me. I couldn't remember a moment like that ever happening during my marriage. This very special man had brought joy into my home. I fell in love with Mike that day. Four years later we were married. Eventually, the people who'd tried to talk us out of marrying, insisting that the age difference was too great, or that he was too young to be saddled with a ready-made family, admitted they were wrong. We adore one another, and I still blush sometimes when I look at him across the table. Whenever anyone asks, "How long have you two been married?" our standard answer is, "Not nearly long enough."

In response to my ex-husband's parting words, I would now say, "You were right. No man in his right mind would want me. But who needs a man in his right mind when a wonderful guy is crazy in love with me?"

Look at us now, I thought, turning away from the view and heading upstairs to get the laundry baskets. The kids are all grown and doing well and we live in our dream home.

When we had our home built, we fully expected to share it with one or more of our parents someday. But it wasn't Rodger we had in mind when we first talked about it.

The year 2002 began as an exciting year for us. We went to Florida for my mother's surprise seventy-fifth birthday party. A New Year's baby, she always loved a big celebration and that one seemed to please her more than most. She held court in the center of the large hall, laughing and opening her many gifts. She flirted and flashed her middle finger as she deemed appropriate. Mike was the recipient of both as the evening progressed. He loved it.

When she'd first entered the room, I was shocked by how frail she looked. She was too thin and her skin had a pale, ashy cast. She appeared to have aged years since I had seen her only a few months before. But she blossomed as the evening wore on and seemed fine when we left for home a few days later.

Mike and I held hands during most of the flight. We were enjoying our empty nest, and the quick trip to Florida would be the beginning of the fun we had planned.

Mike's parents were talking about moving to Virginia to be closer to us and to Mike's brother, Dan, and his family. I was looking forward to having them close by.

A few days later, as we walked through our home-in-progress, we talked about our aging parents and how the day was coming when they'd need someone to care for them. We agreed that when they needed help, we would bring them into our home. At the time, we assumed it would be one of our mothers. We even discussed the possibility it could be both of them for a while. My parents had divorced a long time ago and my father had disappeared into a new life. No one had heard from him in years. Rodger was fifteen years older than his wife, Shirley, and in addition to his nervous condition he'd had cancer and open-heart surgery. There was no reason to think that either man would live with us.

In February, the reason for my mother's frail appearance was identified. She was diagnosed with non-Hodgkin lymphoma. During the long weeks of her illness I made several trips back and forth to be at her side along with my sister and brothers.

It was during one of her better periods, when I went home for a while to be with Mike and to take care of some things at work, that the call came from Pittsburgh. Shirley had died suddenly of a heart attack. Eight weeks later, my mother passed away quietly, surrounded by her family.

We were nearly overcome with sadness. But, even as we struggled to cope with our personal losses and comfort each other, we never wavered in our convictions. As soon as anyone posed the question, "What's going to happen to Rodger?" we responded by saying, "He's coming to live with us."

The first several weeks he was with us sped by in a blur of packing and moving into the new house and getting used to one another. We made the best of our first Christmas in our new home but our joy was tempered with sorrow. Mike spent hours baking cookies using Shirley's holiday recipes. I placed my mother's jaunty dancing Santa on the mantle and dusted off the wax choirboy that used to be part of a set of five. I smiled at his perpetually dirty face, grimy from years of being wrapped in newsprint and packed in a box between holidays. When my sister and brothers and I went through Mom's things, we divvied up the set, each taking the one he or she liked best.

Rodger decided it was his job to decorate the tree. As soon as

Mike had the lights up, he went to work. With the utmost care he lifted each ornament out of its box and hung it right next to the previous one. When he had finished, all the ornaments were clumped together in the top third of the tree. We let it go, content to have him participate.

When the holiday was over, we breathed a sigh of relief. We knew things would be better in the new year. Little did we know that in a few short weeks our lives would change dramatically and we'd be tested in ways we couldn't begin to imagine—and it all started with a party.

"Mom, I think something is wrong with Grampy."

Kelly and her friend Ashley were circulating among the guests, pouring wine and refreshing snack trays while I enjoyed the company of friends and showed off my new house.

I had let Rodger know that a lot of people would be coming so he wouldn't be startled by the presence of strangers.

"Do I have to go?"

"Not if you don't want to."

I wasn't surprised when he said he'd rather not attend.

"It's okay," I reassured him. "No one will bother you. If it gets too noisy, just let me know and we'll tone it down."

"Don't worry about me," he said. "I like to be alone."

I hadn't seen anyone going upstairs unescorted, and the music level was low so I didn't think anyone was disturbing him.

"Do you think I should go up and check on him?" I asked.

"Yes, he's acting funny."

"What does that mean? How is he acting funny?"

"He's hiding by the top of the stairs, and he keeps tiptoeing over to the railing and looking over."

"He's just trying to see what's going on. You know he's shy. He doesn't want to come down but he wants to see who's here."

"No that's not it. He looks like he's mad or scared or something. His eyes look funny."

Neither young woman was particularly skittish, the two of them experiencing more than their share of rowdy fun and adventure throughout high school and as college roommates. Both had a great deal of affection for Grampy, as they called him, so I felt that their reaction to whatever was going on warranted my attention. Taking a small step back to allow for a wider view of the second floor, I scanned the doorway to his room and then over toward the adjacent bathroom.

"I don't see him," I said.

"He's up there," Kelly insisted.

Again I surveyed the upper floor and didn't see him. I was beginning to lose patience with the two of them.

Ashley pointed. "There he is."

It was as if the scene before me was playing out in a movie. The clink of glasses and hum of easy banter faded into the background as my attention focused on the shadowy figure above.

Rodger was up there all right. His body was plastered against the wall, fingers splayed, as if in an effort to make himself disappear into the background. Clearly he did not want to be seen. Seconds ticked by slowly as I waited to see what he'd do next.

"Do you see him?" Kelly whispered.

"I see him."

Looking quickly left and then right, he tiptoed to the railing and peeked over. I could see what my daughter meant. Something about him seemed different. His usual flat expression was gone, his head quickly darting from side to side as he took note of each person in the room below. His eyes widened in shock when he settled on me and realized I was looking back at him.

"What are you doing?" I called up to him. "Do you want to come down and join us?"

"No," he answered brusquely, quickly backing away from the railing and into the room behind him, closing the door.

"What's up with that? That's not like Grampy," Ashley said.

"It's okay," I repeated, hoping to reassure both young women and help shake off my own unease. "He's usually in bed by now. He was probably half asleep, forgot about the party, and wondered what was going on."

I couldn't gauge what effect my words were having on them, but I was doing a pretty good job of convincing myself—right up until the moment the door slowly began to open and one aged hand emerged, feeling its way along the wall. Fascinated, I watched as he quietly eased himself through the narrow opening and again braced his body up against the wall. Anxiously, he scanned the rooms below, searching for someone or something.

What is he looking for?

Puzzled by his odd behavior, I started up the stairs, but before I reached the third step, he spotted me and made a beeline for his bedroom.

"Goodnight," I called out as he scurried into the room and firmly closed the door.

Although unsettled by what I'd seen, I put a smile on my face and went back to my guests, hoping that he had seen enough to ease his mind.

Despite Rodger's odd behavior, the party was a complete success. Mike arrived home just as the last guests pulled out of the driveway. He helped me tidy up. He thanked me again for not insisting that he stay for what we both acknowledged was a "chick party." In a couple of weeks, he'd invite his friends over for burgers and football for the male version of a good housewarming, and I was as fine with that event as he was with mine.

Stifling a yawn of sudden fatigue, I told him about his father's conduct during the party. He suggested that, as odd as it looked to us, it probably seemed perfectly reasonable to someone as introverted as his father, allowing him to check things out without having to interact with people. I convinced myself that what I thought was a suspicious look in his eyes was merely an illusion caused the shadows on the upstairs landing.

Considering that he'd lost his wife of almost forty years, been uprooted from his home. and endured two moves within a matter of months, a little odd behavior was to be expected. All in all, he had handled everything very well. He was determined to be as independent as possible, taking responsibility for counting out his daily medications and filling up his weekly pill box. He kept his room tidy and insisted on taking his daily walks by himself. After dining with us a few evenings, he announced that he'd prefer to have his meals on his own schedule. As that had been the first time he'd asserted himself in any way since moving in with us, we took it as a good sign.

"Take what you want. I'll eat what's leftover," he'd always say. "I don't eat much."

Despite our assurances that there was plenty of food, he'd take only a teaspoonful of each dish, making sure that Mike had his fill before going back for more.

Frequently, we'd hear him foraging in the kitchen after we went to bed and find dishes in the sink in the morning. It broke our hearts to think of him going hungry at mealtime, waiting patiently for an opportunity to eat leftovers. I showed him how to make some simple dishes and how to use the stove and the microwave. We spent a few evenings practicing. It wasn't exactly new to him; he just needed to learn his way around a strange kitchen and get used to the knobs and dials on unfamiliar appliances. Soon he was quite content in his role as cook, and Mike and I were reassured that he was getting enough to eat. .

As willing as I was to accommodate him whenever possible, there was one thing I was determined to change. He had a habit of compartmentalizing the refrigerator and cupboards into sections containing "his food" and "our food." The idea of claiming a chicken leg or a slice of cake as one's own didn't make sense to me. As far as I'm concerned, family members share. When you're hungry, you go to the refrigerator, scout around to see what's there, and make a sandwich or prepare a plate. Not Rodger.

He wouldn't take anything without asking, "Is this for Michael or for me?"

When we'd reply, "It's for anyone who wants it," he'd look puzzled for a few seconds and ask again, "Can I eat this or is it for Michael?"

"It's for you if you want it," we'd say and then watch as he gently placed whatever it might be in his compartment of the refrigerator to enjoy later.

After going around and around on this for weeks, I was about to give in and accept the fact that at 76 years old, he wasn't going to change, when I realized another aspect of this quirk was causing him a great deal of stress.

Mike's mother always kept her cupboards and freezer well stocked. A large Italian woman who liked to cook, she was prepared for any contingency. And if you ever expressed a preference for a certain dish, she made sure she always had the ingredients on hand to make it for you. When she died, the small portable freezer she kept stocked for emergencies was full to the brim with everything from ground meat to pie shells. When we packed Rodger's things for the move to Virginia, we brought the freezer with us. In his mind, the food that came from his house became his responsibility. Cementing this belief was the fact that while the three of us were crammed into a tiny apartment waiting for the new house to be completed, we'd had to put the freezer in Rodger's bedroom.

I'd noticed him rearranging boxes of hamburgers and cans of juice in the freezer a few times and wondered what he was trying to do. I could hear him mumbling softly to himself, but it was never loud enough to be understood. He continued this habit of taking inventory even after we moved the freezer into the garage at the new house. He'd bring me something and ask what it was and how to prepare it. Since many of the things were microwaveable, he'd heat them up for lunch or dinner, paying little notice to what he was eating. A meal of French toast sticks and broccoli seemed to satisfy him just as much as a plate of reheated lasagna.

One Saturday afternoon when I was relaxing on the overstuffed loveseat enjoying a good book and a glass of local wine, he came over and stood quietly in front of me.

"What's this meat?" he asked when I looked up from my reading.

"It's a ham."

"Show me how to cook it." He started rocking side to side, his voice trembling.

A bit irritated at being interrupted, I tried to wave him off. "I'll show you another time. I'm reading now," I said softly.

"I have to cook it," he insisted. "I have to eat it before it goes bad." The rocking increased as he spoke and his hand began to tremble. "Can't waste, have to eat it," he mumbled. His normally droopy shoulders slumped even more as he turned to walk away.

"What's wrong?" I asked, putting my book aside.

"There's too much food. I can't eat it all. It's going to go bad. Oh no, can't waste it. Oh no …"

"Don't worry," I reassured him. "You don't have to cook that right now. It's frozen. It will last for a long time that way."

"It's too much," he insisted. "I can't eat all that food. It's going to go bad."

"I'll cook the ham another day, then we can all eat it. You don't have to eat that by yourself."

"No?" he asked.

"No that's too much for one person. That's for a family to eat."

"But the box, the cold box, it's full."

"You mean the freezer?"

"Yes, the freezer, it's too much."

"You're right, that's too much for you. We can share."

"Yeah," he tried to smile. "We can all eat."

The relief he felt was visible as the tension left his face. I gently took the meat from him and went to the kitchen. Soon the aroma of baked ham filled the room. While Rodger napped and Michael cut the grass, I transferred everything from his cold box to the freezer compartments of our two refrigerators. The next time Mike's brother Dan and his family came to visit, we sent the small freezer home with them.

What will he come up with next? I wondered.

Chapter 3

"Oh my God, Mike. Your father is crazy."

That afternoon I had received a copy of Rodger's medical records from the VA hospital in Pittsburgh. As a 100% disabled veteran, he received all his medical care there before coming to live with us. Another complete set had been sent to the VA hospital in Martinsburg, WV, where he'd receive treatment from now on.

Shocked by what I'd discovered among the hundreds of pages of medical records I'd just begun to read, I had spoken without thinking.

"What do you mean he's crazy? Why do you say that?"

"According to this," I said, tapping the page, "he was diagnosed as paranoid schizophrenic in 1949. He's been hospitalized for treatment several times since then."

I handed my husband a page from the pile of documents I held in my hands. Dated April 17, 1987, it read:

> The patient is a 60-year-old, disabled, white, married male of Italian extraction who served in the Army and has a 100% service-connected disability rating and who is presently admitted for bizarre behavior and poor compliance with neuroleptic medications.
>
> The patient came to the Mental Hygiene Clinic in August of 1985 with multiple hospitalizations for a schizophrenia illness in the past. The patient's psychiatric history began with a psychotic episode in the early part of 1949 while in the service in Italy. At that time he was apparently confused, had hallucinated, and was delusional. He was given insulin and shock therapy and his psychotic symptoms went into remission. He, however, continued to have some difficulties and remained a resident of the VAMC in Chillicothe, OH.

He was discharged from Chillicothe, OH, in February of 1960. At that time his diagnosis was schizophrenic reaction, paranoid type, chronic. He was thought to have a marked schizoid personality due in part to early loss of his father due to the father's migration to the United States, and experiences as a youth in Italy during World War II. … After his discharge from the hospital, the patient was able to begin working, and sometime shortly after discharge, the patient returned to Italy with his mother, where he required evaluation for his "depression." It was recommended that the patient return to the United States for treatment. In 1964, the patient returned to the United States, was followed in the Mental Hygiene Clinic Associated with the VAMC (Veterans Association Medical Center), and obtained employment as a janitor for the post office and married. The patient married a woman who was younger than he who had a 7-year-old son. He subsequently had a son with this wife. The patient functioned well until 1979 when he required psychiatric hospitalization at Braddock. The patient subsequently retired on disability.

Mike and I were aware that his father had been hospitalized several times since then for his "nerves." Yet, in the fifteen years before he came to live with us, no one had ever mentioned paranoia or schizophrenia as a reason for his behavior.

"Did you know about this?" I asked.

"No I didn't," Mike answered, concern evident in his expression.

"How can that be? Didn't your mother ever say anything to you?"

"No. All she said was that he had a nervous condition from being in the war. Honest, honey, I didn't know."

Looking into my husband's beautiful brown eyes, I knew he was being honest. His mother had explained his father's early retirement and introverted behavior using the same words when I first met him. It's the same story some family members still believe to be true, although I later discovered that a few people were told he had a metal plate in his head due to a war wound, I knew of no one who was ever told the true nature of his illness.

"So what are you thinking?" Mike asked after a few moments of silence.

"I'm thinking we're in for a more interesting time than we thought and ..."

"And what? Are you afraid of him now?"

"No. As long as he's medicated, he'll be fine."

"Then what is it?"

"I think I need to get some training."

"What kind of training?"

I pointed to the pile of records. "Based on this information, and some stuff you haven't seen yet about his medical problems, and the fact that he is almost eighty years old, I want to get some basic medical training. I want to make sure I'll know how to assess his vital signs, monitor his medication, etc. There may come a time when he'll need daily injections of some sort. I think it's best we be prepared for whatever may come. What do you think?"

"I think," my husband responded, "that I love you very much and that I'm very lucky to have you—and so is my dad."

Even as I set aside the thick sheaf of papers I'd been reading and settled into Mike's arms, I wondered if I'd be up to the challenges ahead.

"I sure hope so," I prayed, not realizing I'd spoken the words out loud.

"I do," Mike answered, misunderstanding my comment. "I really, really believe that. And don't worry. Now that he's with us and he doesn't have to worry about taking care of my mom, he'll be able to relax and take things easy for a change. Being here with us will be good for him. You'll see." And then he kissed me, pushing all thoughts of paranoia and psychotic episodes out of my head for the evening.

Later, as I whispered one more silent prayer before drifting off to sleep, I heard the faint squeaking of the floorboards. Rodger was out there, pacing and listening.

Over the next few weeks, Mike's prediction seemed to be coming true. Because Rodger was so introverted and so reluctant to impose on us in any way, we decided to furnish the spare room next to his bedroom as a sitting room. In it we placed a sofa, a big green leather recliner, a television, and an end table to hold his ever-present glass of water. Just a few steps away was his full bathroom. With the exception of a kitchen, he now had his own small efficiency apartment on the second floor.

"This house is a dream come true. It couldn't be better," he said one day.

Mike beamed. "Wow, did you hear that?"

My response was a smile as big as his. We both thought he was settling in well. We had no reason to suspect he was planning to move out.

It was Mike's turn to take his father to see his psychiatrist. I was in the middle of a busy workweek, typing away on a report with a rapidly approaching deadline, when he called to let me know they were back from the doctor.

"How did it go?" I asked, fully expecting to hear good news.

"Well, not quite as expected." Mike hesitated.

"What's wrong? Is he sick?" Immediately, I started taking inventory in my mind. I had completed a basic medical assisting course and knew his blood pressure and heart rate were good. He was eating well. He didn't have a cold or a fever or any signs of flu. What could it be?

"No, he's not sick. He told his psychiatrist that he didn't want to go home. Apparently, he's been thinking about this for a while."

"Why?" I asked after a few moments of shocked silence.

"He doesn't want to be a burden. He says it's too much work for us."

"Oh boy."

"Yes, and he said we both work, he's alone, and he might have an emergency."

"What do we do now?"

"We can't force him to stay, and he is a hundred percent disabled. They'll take him if he needs a place to go."

"He doesn't need a place to go," I insisted. "He'll die in a place like that."

"I know," Mike agreed. "I feel the same way. Now we have to convince him of that. They've arranged for a meeting with a social worker at the hospital, and I'm going to talk to the guy before we go and convince him to work with us to assure Dad that he's better off at home."

When we got to the meeting later in the month, the social worker quietly spoke with Rodger. He asked about his living conditions, the food, if he was treated well. Was he unhappy or afraid? But even after he reassured everyone that he was not unhappy and the home he lived in was beautiful, "the best house I ever had," it still took a lot of convincing to get him to agree to stay.

"When the time comes that you really need us, Mr. Carducci, we'll be here for you." The counselor spoke gently but firmly, placing a hand on his shoulder. "You earned that right by serving your country, and we won't let you down. For now, we have to take care of men and women who don't have a good home to go to or family to be with. Okay, sir?"

"Okay," he sighed, rising and reaching for the door. "Let's go home."

All our efforts to convince him that home was the best place for him had not been totally convincing but, for the moment at least, he was willing to accept it.

Rodger was quiet most of the way home. I thought he'd fallen asleep, until we turned onto our street and I heard him talking to himself.

"They told me that I could come back if I needed. It don't make sense. If there's no room, there's no hope."

Sometimes I still hear those words: If there's no room, there's no hope. But I no longer believe he was referring to the hospital. Devastating illness was again beginning to fill his mind with so many dark thoughts that the light of hope had dimmed within him. Yet, despite the difficulties that were to come, and my moments of weakness in dealing with them, I knew in my heart that his indomitable spirit kept a small, but incredibly strong, spark of hope burning even through the worst of his problems.

Chapter 4

"I called 911."

Rodger was seated at the kitchen table, his hand resting gently on the phone in front of him. He spoke up as I turned on the water to rinse my teacup before leaving for work. I wasn't sure I'd heard him correctly.

"Hmm?"

"I called 911."

"When?"

"Three or four minutes ago."

"Why?"

"I wanted to see if it works here. In Pittsburgh, you call 911 and the cops come. Sometimes an ambulance comes."

"Are you serious? What did you tell them?"

"Nothing. I hung up. Then a lady called. She said, 'Did you call 911?' I told her yes. I had to check if it works."

"You're only supposed to call if there's a real emergency," I reminded him.

"Yeah, call 911 for emergency. Just like Pittsburgh. But the lady, she called back."

I shook my head, wondering what he'd think of next, hoping now that he'd verified that it worked, he wouldn't feel the need to try it again.

"Don't call them anymore, okay? Unless it's an emergency. Somebody might need them and they'll be talking to you instead. Promise me."

"No, I won't call no more."

What a way to start the day, I thought, opening the kitchen door and pressing the button for the garage door opener. As it began to rise, I saw the tires and bumper of a car in front of the opening. Then I saw the familiar brown paint used on the local sheriff's cars.

Standing beside it was a deputy, speaking quietly into the radio attached to the loop on his shoulder. "Everything appears quiet," he was saying.

I stepped out to greet him and explained about my father-in-law and his call to make sure 911 works in Virginia. The deputy was very understanding, and when Rodger joined us in the driveway to tell his side of the story, the man listened patiently and reassured him that 911 worked fine around there, and that if he needed assistance, it would be dispatched quickly. Then with a tip his hat and a, "Have a nice day," he was gone.

"I told the lady not to send anyone," Rodger insisted.

"She had to," I said. "When they get a call and someone hangs up, they have to check it out. What if you were having a heart attack or a stroke and got confused?"

"I told her everything was okay. She's crazy for calling the cops."

"No. She's not crazy. What if a bad guy was in there with a gun, and you tried to call and he caught you and made you say everything was fine. She has to tell the police so they can check. So don't call anymore, please.

"Okay, but that lady is crazy."

Someone's crazy, I thought as I pulled out of the driveway and pointed my car toward work. *But it's not that lady, and it could very well end up being me if this kind of thing keeps up.*

Once I had my work organized for the day, I called Mike and shared my little morning adventure with him.

"No way!" He laughed.

"Oh yes. And he thinks the 911 lady is crazy for calling the cops on him."

Even while we were joking about it, we recognized that this, like the request to live in a nursing home, was another sign that Rodger did not feel comfortable being alone in that big house all day.

"I think we better set aside some time later on to talk about what we can do to relieve his anxiety."

"Yes," Mike agreed. "It's not fair to him to let things continue this way."

Although we suspected what the solution had to be, Mike and I spent many hours over the next few days talking and planning and exploring options before finally admitting that it was time I quit my job.

Once the decision was made, Mike sat quietly for several moments, a thoughtful look on his face. I wondered if he was secretly worried that the financial burden of losing my paycheck was going to have a greater impact than I thought. We had just taken on a brand-new mortgage, and his commute had almost doubled with the move, adding additional expenses for gas and parking.

"What's wrong? Is it the finances you're concerned about?"

"No, as far as money goes we'll be fine. We're very lucky in that respect. Yes, we'll lose your paycheck, but my dad has his disability check each month. Instead of putting it into a savings account as we have been, we can use part of it to cover the loss of your income."

"What do you think your brother will say about that?"

"I can't see where he can object. We're the ones taking care of my father, and the money will go to his support. I don't think it will be a problem. We all know that the best place for my dad is here with us. It's clean and safe and we care about him. This is where he should be."

"I agree completely. So, if it's not the money, what's bothering you?"

"I feel so guilty."

"About what?" I asked, confused as all hell by that response.

"About asking you to quit your job to take care of my father. It doesn't seem right that you'll be bearing the brunt of his care."

I couldn't help but laugh.

"What's so funny?" Mike tried to smile. "Why are you laughing at me?"

"I'm laughing at the idea of you feeling guilty over this. First, he's not just your father, he's our family. And, second, picture this scenario: I wake up in my beautiful new home and see to it that he takes his meds and has breakfast. Then I run the Swiffer over the hardwood floors before taking the newspaper and my cup of tea out onto the deck. If I finish the paper before I'm ready to go in, I'll be forced to look at the view. Yes, my darling, feel very guilty about that. In fact, feel so guilty that you put a hot tub on that deck to ease your conscience, and after a really rough day, I'll join you in taking a long, soothing soak."

"Hey, wait a minute." He grinned. "Now that you put it that way, he's my father and maybe I should be the one to sacrifice my job and stay home."

"Too late," I teased back. "The position's been filled. And besides, it never hurts to have a man feel obligated to his wife. Just think of all the great presents you're going to have to buy me to assuage those guilt feelings."

The next day I turned in my two-week notice.

"What are you going to do all day?" my friends and coworkers asked when word got around the office that I was quitting.

"I'm worried about what will happen to you," my daughter confided. "It's not going to be easy to be home alone all the time."

"Are you sure you want to do this?" was a question Mike and I heard over and over. "It's not going to be easy, you know."

My standard response to people who posed those questions was, "I'm setting an example for my children."

It usually took a few seconds for the message behind those words to sink in, but when it did people began to smile. Sooner or later, they realized, we all reach the point where we need help. When it's my turn, I hope my family will be there for me.

My daughter used to say, "Mom, I'll never put you in a nursing home."

And I'd tell her, "But I want you to. I don't ever want to be a burden."

After seeing my mother deteriorate rapidly after a brief stay in a nursing home while battling her long illness, and hearing stories from others about the inconsistent care their elderly relatives receive in those places, I now tell my kids, "Put the addition on the house, I'm coming."

So, yes, I was setting an example for my children, one that was set by my aunt Pat who cared for my grandfather for several years after he developed dementia. Then she and her daughter tended my uncle Jim at home when he was dying from cancer. Even Rodger spent many years helping his mother during the time she lived in an assisted living facility. He was at her side when she passed away at the age of 102. Family takes care of family. Now that Rodger needed someone, Mike and I were determined to be there for him.

Several weeks later, on a picture-perfect morning just like the one I had described to my husband, I splashed a dollop of fat-free cream into my mug of tea, added a half-teaspoon of sugar, and opened the sliding glass door onto the deck. Even though I no longer had to cope with the morning rush hour to make it to an office on time, I still got up at seven each morning, showered, and put on makeup. Instead of business attire I wore jeans and T-shirts; and, instead of matching my shoes to my dress, I went barefoot around the house. But I still wanted to look presentable as I went about my day. At 5'7" and 130-135 pounds, depending on the day, I'd finally come to like the way I looked. Never considered beautiful, I was capable of being pretty with some effort—and on most days I made the effort. For a woman in my fifties and the grandmother of four, I'd done well in maintaining what I had.

One of my earliest memories is of my mother brushing my big sister's hair before school. I couldn't have been more than four at the time. My sister Catherine, called Kitty, was two years older and I idolized her. I watched as our mother ran the brush through Kitty's long hair, listening as she told her how she'd grow up to be a real beauty, and boys would flock around her and take her on dates.

"You look like me," our mother said. "And with your strawberry blonde hair, everyone will notice you. You'll go to parties and dances and have lots of boyfriends."

"Me too," I said.

"No not you," Mom answered. "You look like your aunt. If you work at it, you can be cute, and if you're nice, some of the boys who hang around your sister will go out with you after she breaks their hearts."

I remembered being told that my hair was "dirty blonde," not strawberry like my sister's, and that I'd be skinny and not fill out like Kitty would. Mom also said that I wouldn't be as smart as Kitty. She was right about the boys and the dates, but she was wrong about the rest. Maybe my sister started out smarter, and maybe she didn't, but I always got better grades than she did. That could have been because Kitty was always flirting and going out while I stayed home and studied, but it didn't really matter in the long run. Life didn't end up the way Mom had predicted for either of us. Yet, despite her poor track record in making predictions, her words had a profound effect on her two little girls and the way they came to see themselves.

Momentarily distracted from my thoughts, I watched through the glass doors as Rodger shuffled into the kitchen, opened the pantry, and retrieved a dishtowel from its hook just inside the door. He'd already eaten his breakfast and gone out to get the morning paper. He opened the dishwasher and methodically started to put everything away, one piece at time. Grasping a plate with both hands, he lifted it out of the rack, turned with deliberation, and walked to the cupboard. Watching in amazement at the concentrated effort of every movement, I imagined I could hear the familiar *swish* of his bedroom slippers dragging across the hardwood floor with each step. With studied care he lifted the plate, set it firmly in place on top of the stack, and rested for a second before heading back to repeat the process. It would take almost twenty minutes to put everything away. I could have done it in three or four, but this was his job; he'd made that very clear right from the beginning.

"I do it," he told me the first morning he was with us. "I can do it. In Pittsburgh, I did it for Shirley."

Many times I sat at my mother-in-law's kitchen table and observed her watching him remove one load of dishes to make room for the next. Heaven forbid if he should try to put something where it didn't belong.

"Damn it, Rodger! How many times do I have to tell you that the spatula goes in the drawer under the microwave? Don't you dare put that bowl with the blue ones. It goes on the top shelf with the clear set. Put that knife in the right way. Do you want me to cut my hand off reaching in there?"

Her constant nitpicking set my nerves on edge. I wondered how he put up with the constant nagging, and how she could stand being so agitated all the time. To me, it didn't seem worth the stress, and Michael agreed. If Rodger put something where it didn't normally go, we never mentioned it.

"Treasure hunt," one of us would declare while searching for the beaters for the electric mixer or a wooden spoon. It became a regular game in our kitchen, one of the quirky little things that made our house a home. But, every now and then, something got misplaced never to be found. Most often it was the lids to plastic storage bowls, but sometimes it was a small bowl, a spatula, or even a measuring cup.

For the longest time I couldn't figure out where he was putting them. I'd do a thorough search of the drawers and cabinets and come up with nothing. And then one day I was talking to a relative who had spent months visiting my in-laws. She told me that he used to get in a lot of trouble at home for throwing away the lids to his wife's Tupperware. If the drawer for the lids was full and he couldn't find room for one more, he figured it wasn't needed and he'd throw it away. I thought about the frequent disarray in my kitchen drawers and how, sometimes, I had to maneuver things around to get something to fit. All of a sudden the mystery of the missing kitchen stuff was solved. I had to laugh. How utterly efficient he was. If there's no room, it means you have too much and it's time to get rid of something. I couldn't help but think maybe more people should do things his way.

He was reaching for one of the last two cups in the rack when he froze in place. Still half bent over, his arm extended toward the cup, he stopped moving for several seconds. From his pose he might have been an oversized child caught up in a game of statues on a warm summer night. But this was no game. Very slowly, while his body remained rigid, his head began to move from side to side, increasing in speed as the seconds ticked by.

Oh no, there he goes again. I set my cup on the table, reaching for the door at the same time.

"Rodger!" I called, moving toward him quickly. "Rodger," I said again, reaching him and gently touching his shoulder. His head had started moving rapidly up and down and from side to side with increasing force.

"Rodger, what are you doing?"

As soon as my words registered, the motion stopped. His body straightened and he looked around, his eyes blinking rapidly.

"What?" he said, a slightly defensive tone in his voice.

"You were shaking your head again. Are you all right?"

"I'm okay. Sometimes I shake, that's all."

Sometimes you shake, I thought. *But that's not all.* There had to be a reason for the increasing number of spasms or seizures or whatever they were, and I was determined to find out what it was. Every time he saw one of his doctors, I reported the headshaking and the hand tremors and the involuntary shudders that hit him from time to time. No one had been able to explain it. And the odd movements weren't the only thing that concerned me.

When he wasn't downstairs with us, he was almost always outside his room ... lurking. The odd behavior that first manifested itself the night of the housewarming party had become a constant in our lives. Every evening, and frequently during the day, we heard him walking back and forth on the upstairs hallway. When we looked up, he was either peering over the banister or huddled up against the wall, trying to avoid being seen. I'd go upstairs and find him facing the wall in the large spare bedroom, his arms crossed loosely as he tried to appear nonchalant. I knew he'd darted in there when he heard me coming. Although I knew the old man was harmless and it was only his odd way of being part of things, I found it creepy being watched in my own home.

With a smile, Rodger insisted he was fine. "When you get old, you shake sometimes," was all he had to say on the subject. He carefully lifted the last of the cups from the rack and gently put it in its proper place. "I'll go for a walk now."

The longer the headshaking went on, the stronger the movements became. Fearing he was causing unseen damage to himself, I reached for the phone and made another appointment for him so see a doctor. This time I got lucky. They could fit him in to see his primary care physician on the same day he was scheduled to see his psychiatrist. Perhaps one of them would finally be able to figure this out.

"Mr. Carducci, how are you today?" his psychiatrist asked.

"Good."

"Any problems at home?"

"No. I can't sleep too good. But sometimes I sleep during the day."

The doctor looked at me. Both of us heard the same words every time he entered this office. Just as he had said the same words to every other doctor he'd seen in the past thirty years. Despite the fact that he napped regularly and slept soundly through the night most of the time, Rodger believed he had chronic insomnia. Every time he saw a doctor and every time someone asked him how he was, he said the same thing.

"I don't sleep much."

An excerpt from his medical records dated 03/03/92 reads as follows:

Mr. Carducci is a 65-year-old white, married, 100% service-connected for schizophrenic reaction, paranoid male vet seen for a scheduled visit.

The vet complains that he is continuously feeling anxious, depressed, and irritable because "I cannot sleep very well, I can only sleep 3-5 hours per night."

... He is anxious and mildly depressed-looking but denies that he is suicidal or homicidal at this time. ... The vet says he is not going outside very much because "the people make me so nervous and uncomfortable." ... The intellectual capacity appears to be of below average. The insight is somewhat limited and also judgment appears to be questionable at times.

Diagnosis: Schizoaffective disorder.

Treatment Plan:

1. Supportive counseling on each visit for chronic mood and thinking disorders.

2. Continue amitriptyline 75 mg HS and Thorazine 50 mg HS. to control thinking and mood disturbances.

3. Return to MHC in three months for follow-up or may call as needed.

He'd even been tested in a sleep clinic. The results indicated that he fell asleep quickly and stayed that way for seven hours before waking and declaring he'd been up all night. Despite evidence to the contrary, Rodger continued to insist that he did not sleep.

"Do you sleep during the day?" the doctor asked.

"Sometimes," he admitted.

"Maybe you should try to stay up during the day and sleep at night."

"I have to sleep when it comes," he insisted. "Sometimes I don't close an eye all night. People tell me I snore. They say I sleep. I don't know. For years I never sleep."

Giving up on that issue once again, the doctor turned to me. "How is he otherwise?"

"I'm worried. He's having the headshaking spells more often, and they last longer than they did when they started. Sometimes he freezes in place when he's walking across a room. He wiggles and shakes his shoulders when he's trying to eat too. Sometimes it looks like he's dancing in his chair."

The doctor turned his attention back to Rodger, observing him as he questioned him. "Are you feeling depressed?" he asked.

"No."

"Are you feeling like you want to hurt yourself or others?"

"No. Everything's nice. Nice house. Nice food. I couldn't ask for better. I worry about them, that's all. I don't want to be no trouble. If I can stay in the hospital, I don't mind. I'm used to it. I stayed in the hospital for thirteen years. Most of it in an open ward. I did details. Wash the floor, clean needles. Something to do, you know."

"Other people need to be in the hospital more than you do," the doctor reminded him. "You have a good home with your family. Some men have no one."

Turning back to me, the doctor said, "I see some tongue movements and other symptoms of what's called Tardive Dyskinesia. It's caused by the long-term use of antipsychotic drugs, such as the ones he's taken for so many years. It can manifest in involuntary movements of the lips, face, tongue, and body. We can try adjusting his medication to see if we can relieve some of the symptoms, but we can't cure it. Also, finding the right dose can be difficult. What you're seeing can be caused by either too much or too little medication. I'm going to decrease his dosage a bit and have you bring him back next month so I can see how he's doing. If you have any problems in the meantime, let me know."

An hour later, his primary care doctor checked him over and declared his problems to be psych related and told me to stick with the advice his psychiatrist offered.

"Of course, if he gets worse, you can bring him in and we'll check him over," he said, leading me toward the door.

I didn't feel comforted by the words of either doctor, and it didn't help matters that during all the time we had been in with them, Rodger had not exhibited any of the symptoms I was concerned about.

"When do we have to go back?" he asked as we walked to the car.

"In a month," I told him, checking the new prescription I picked up at the hospital pharmacy.

"Why do we have to come back so much? In Pittsburgh, I go every six months."

"We're trying to find out why your head shakes and you get stuck sometimes."

"When you get old, you shake, that's all," he insisted.

"You're not that old. You're only seventy-six, and your mother lived to be over one hundred. Her head didn't shake like that."

"Yeah, I'm not that ol ...," his words trailed off to nothing as he froze in place and his head began to bob just steps from the car.

"Come on, Rodger." I spoke firmly to rouse him from this latest episode. "Let's get you home."

"Why we have to come back so soon? In Pittsburgh, I only had to go every six months," he repeated.

That evening I started him on the decreased dose of medicine. The following month we went back to report that the symptoms were increasing. The headshaking and twitching were more frequent than before. I mentioned the lurking again and Rodger told the doctor he was just going to the bathroom. I knew that wasn't true, but I didn't know how to make the doctor understand. How many times must I explain that he wasn't just hesitating in a doorway on his way out, and that most people don't sidle along the walls on their way to the toilet?

When the doctors continued to be unconcerned over the next couple of months, I tried to convince myself they were right.

After all, Rodger often did things that didn't make sense at first but proved to be logical enough once he explained them. Like the time I was away and Mike came home from work and noticed something stuck to his father's foot.

"Hold on a minute, you have some plastic tape or something stuck to the bottom of your slipper."

"It's not tape. It's a bread bag."

"Why do you have your foot in a bread bag?"

"I cut my toe," he explained. "I was clipping my toenails and I caught a piece of skin. It was bleeding. I couldn't find a Band-Aid. I didn't want to get blood on the rug. I put the bread in a plastic dish and put my foot in the bag. It's okay. It works."

We laughed at the idea of a foot in bread bag, but Mike and I had to admit that what appeared to be crazy on the surface turned out to be a real lesson in creative problem-solving. We were a bit more open-minded the next time he did something that seemed odd to us.

Every summer Mike plants a small vegetable garden in the back yard. I love summer tomatoes, still warm from the sun, and he takes great pride in bringing them to me. Rodger lived on a farm in Italy as a boy and knew about growing things, so we decided to ask for his help. It would give him something to do besides going for a walk, bringing in the mail, and putting dishes away each day. It would lure him outside and give him a reason to spend time with his son.

Everything was going along fine; the plants were in and growing nicely. Rodger checked on them regularly and watered them as needed. As the fruit grew in size, some of the plants started to bend under the weight, and before Mike had a chance to tie up one to a support stake, one slender stalk broke. Rodger noticed the injured plant on one of his morning trips outside and did what he could to fix the problem. When Mike went out to check on the garden one evening, he discovered that one of the tomato plants was sporting a Band-Aid. Rodger had carefully lifted the broken stalk back into place and wrapped a Band-Aid around the break to hold the pieces together. Then he had retrieved a small stick from the yard and pushed it into the soft earth next to the plant, using blades of grass to tie it gently to the support. Again, what seemed odd at first turned out to be brilliant in its simplicity. That tomato plant grew better and stronger than all the others that year, and the fruit seemed to taste especially sweet.

Unfortunately, what started out as something good quickly turned into an obsession for him. Before long he was checking on the plants several times a day. When Mike went away on a business trip, it got worse. He began to obsess over what might be too much sun, or the possibility of not enough water. I'd look for him, thinking he'd been out walking much longer than usual, and find him on the deck staring down at the plants, watching them grow. He was wearing himself out dragging the heavy hose across the deck and watering not only the little vegetable garden but all the flowers, trees, and bushes in the yard. Several times I had to remind him that he had already watered that day, or stop him from watering after a rain.

"I'm trying to take care of the garden, but I'm not strong like I used to be. When you get old, you're not strong anymore."

"You don't have to do it," I reassured him. "Mike and I can water the plants and pick the vegetables."

"No, I can do it." He stiffened. "A little bit at a time. Not too much at once, that's all."

No matter how hard I tried, I could not convince him that the yard would be fine until Mike returned. I resigned myself to watching over him to make sure he didn't overdo it. Even that turned into a bigger job than expected. It soon became clear that he didn't appreciate being watched and was taking great pains to stay out of my sight, resulting in a rather pathetic game of hide-and-seek each day. I wished I didn't have to monitor him so closely. I understood exactly how he felt, having someone hover over him, watching his every move, but I didn't dare leave him alone in the yard for very long, fearing that he'd get stuck in a headshaking episode and lose track of time. Both of us were greatly relieved when Mike returned and resumed taking care of the garden. It didn't stop Rodger from watching over the plants during the day, but it did allow him to go off duty when Mike came home in the evening.

Besides obsessing over the plants in Mike's absence, Rodger had doubled his surveillance over me. Not only did he peer at me from the stairs each night as I ate dinner and watched TV, he started pacing outside the bedroom door after I went to bed.

The idea of him lurking and pacing out there was so unnerving I started locking the door and making sure both the bedroom and the master bathroom doors were locked when I took a shower. I wasn't really afraid of him but it unnerved me. I'd watched too many spooky movies to feel safe behind a shower curtain. Fortunately, the shower I had now came with a glass door and no one could sneak up on me. Still, I knew if he peeked in while I was in there I'd jump out of my skin in fright before either of us realized what was happening.

I kept a light on all the time and read into the wee hours of the morning whenever Mike was away, falling asleep when dawn began to lighten the sky and I was too exhausted to keep my eyes open any longer.

Looking into the mirror in the morning, I had to admit that now I was the one anxious and mildly depressed-looking. Fortunately, a swift application of concealer under my eyes, and a touch of lipstick and mascara hid most of the ravages of going without sleep. I was doubly glad when Mike came home and I could rest peacefully again. I'd be myself in no time. We were not even close to being able to say that about Rodger.

Chapter 5

"He's getting worse," I told the doctors over the next several visits. First, they'd reduced his antipsychotic drugs, and then increased the dose to a higher one than any he'd been on before. A mood enhancer was added and still nothing changed. Not that I expected it would. It wasn't his mood causing him to freeze in place and behave like a teenaged headbanger at a never-ending concert.

The only good news came from the cardiologist. Rodger had had an artificial valve placed in his heart a few years earlier. He was lucky that the problem was discovered before he had a heart attack. His specialist assured us his heart was good for another twenty years. His primary care doctor was satisfied that his general health was good, despite a mild case of chronic obstructive pulmonary disease, or COPD. Three times a day he took his breathing treatments in his room. He got his flu shot each year and his pneumonia vaccine as scheduled. He ate better than most people, preferring lots of fruits and vegetables to heavy meals, and had stopped eating beef when his heart problem was diagnosed. For a very sick man, his body was holding up very well.

At home his lurking and rocking and snooping continued. Yet through it all, he kept up with his medications. He'd sit at the kitchen table and painstakingly fill out the order forms for refills, and when they came he'd check all the dosages and read all the information material that came with them. He kept a list of all his meds in his wallet and could tell each doctor what he was taking and what it was for. Right on time he'd go to the cupboard to get his medicine. Just like clockwork, every day, three times a day. Or so we thought—until I spotted him putting them into his pocket one day.

I'd been out shopping and was struggling with several grocery bags when I entered the kitchen. "Why didn't you take your pills?

"What?"

"Your medicine. You better take it now."

"I did."

"I saw you put the pills into your pocket. You need to take it on time."

"I take them upstairs. I have to go to the bathroom first."

"Take them now and then you can go to the bathroom."

With a heavy sigh and a scathing glance, reminding me all too well of one of my kids as a chastened teenager, he deliberately took one pill at time, placed it squarely on the middle of his tongue, and washed it down with a drink of water. Then he stuck his tongue out as far as he could to show me it was gone. Still not satisfied with his dramatic performance, he ended it by walking away, muttering under his breath about trust and being able to take care of himself. He looked so much like a kid I had to laugh. It was right about then Mike and I realized that in the circle of life Rodger had reverted to childhood. We started to affectionately refer to him as "Junior" when he acted out.

I often wondered if he'd do better with a more outgoing person. I like people, but it's hard for me to reach out to them. The two of us alone in the house all day made for a lot of quiet time.

"Do you want to go out for a while?"

"Where?"

Over to the senior center. You can meet people your age. Make friends and play cards or something."

"No. I have nothing to say to those people. Leave me alone."

His records clearly indicated his aversion to being with people. We were not about to force him into anything and dropped that idea almost as quickly as it arose. But I did pay attention to his moods. I sat with him at the table while he ate his lunch and his dinner. If he stared down at his plate and ignored me, I'd leave him alone. But if he looked up and started to talk, I stayed and listened as long as he had something to say.

"I always had food when I was hungry and a job when I needed one," he told me one day. "I never thought I'd be able to raise a family," he whispered, tears shining in his dark eyes. "But I was lucky. I was finally able to do it."

"Yes you did," I reassured him. "You raised two fine sons."

Another time he spoke of his life in Italy as a young boy. He told me about an idyllic summer day when he came upon a large tree lush with ripe fruit. He described how he searched the ground for just the right stone and aimed for the best piece, only to have disaster strike when he missed. His eyes scanned the air above him while he remembered how he stood transfixed as the stone fell and hit a passing chicken on the head, killing it instantly. Confused and alarmed about what had just happened, and wondering how to explain a dead chicken to his mother, he placed it on a nearby haystack, hoping a hungry passerby would find it and enjoy a bountiful meal. I like to believe it happened just that way.

Sometimes he spoke of darker times, like when the Gestapo seized their farm and chased him from his home.

"The German soldier kept kicking me in my ass and telling me to move faster. I don't know why I had to hurry," he said, shaking his head. "I was going. No one could stay there and get kicked in the ass for very long."

"You're lucky he didn't shoot you."

He nodded solemnly. "You need luck to survive in this world."

No matter how many times he told the same story, I listened in the hope that as the days passed he'd reveal more of himself. I'd seen pictures of him as young man. He was strikingly handsome, and I was sure a lot of young Italian women noticed him. I hoped to hear of dates and parties and stolen kisses under the moonlight. Nothing like that was ever mentioned. He rarely spoke of interaction with anyone. To listen to him you'd think he'd lived a very solitary life.

From clinical record dated 10-25-50:

> … Diagnosis: Schizophrenic reaction, paranoid type, chronic, moderate.
>
>   1. External precipitating stress: Not apparent.

2. Predisposition: Marked schizoid personality in childhood and youth. Early loss of father due to migration to the U.S.; experiences in youth with unpleasant aliens (Fascist and Nazi); and changes in cultural pattern with resultant language difficulty.

Present state of service-connected disability: Unchanged.

Despite having a brother he loved and respected, a sister he spoke of with pride, and having devoted many years to caring for his mother after his father's death, he was truly alone most of his life, trapped inside a damaged mind and struggling to build a life as best he could. He was twenty-four years old when those notes were placed in his file. If anyone were to read the notes his present psychiatrist wrote when we left the hospital on any given day, it would still say:

Present state of service-connected disability: Unchanged.

I wished I could say the same, that he had remained unchanged since coming to live with us. But that wasn't true. I was desperate to find a way to get him back to where he was when he came to us, or find out what was making him worse and figure out how to deal with it.

He was having several episodes a day of headshaking and trembling. They came so often I stayed close enough to help pull him out of it during a meal. I didn't dare allow him to go out for a walk, but he rarely asked anymore. He seemed to have lost interest in going outside, except to get the mail, and then he'd come right back in and go back to his room. It was a chore to get him to take a shower and he often smelled bad.

"People in the old country don't wash like people here," he insisted one morning when I reminded him again that it had been several days since he'd bathed. "Too much soap is bad for your skin. They take a bath once a week, every two weeks, once a month maybe."

"That was fifty years ago and things have changed. They have showers and better soap and they wash every day."

"No. Nothing's changed. You don't know nothing about Italy."

Seeing how agitated he was, I backed off on that tactic. "Maybe I don't know about Italy, but I do know about America, and here we wash our bodies and our hair regularly. You don't have to take a shower every day but you do have to be clean. Right now you stink. Go take a shower."

"My mother died and my wife died. I can do what I want," he shouted.

"I'm sorry your mother died and your wife died," I shouted back. "And I know you don't like being told what to do. You can do what you want but you have to do it clean! You smell bad and it's not good for you. Now go take a shower or I'll wash you myself."

A few minutes later I heard his shower running, and shortly after that I saw him walking to his room, his naked backside still glistening with water droplets. I had never seen him do that before and couldn't help but laugh. If he was deliberately mooning me to show his displeasure, I didn't care. I was also very relieved he hadn't called my bluff. I doubted I could successfully bathe an agitated adult man, no matter how old.

He was quiet the rest of the day. Even his television, usually on all day and most of the night, was mute. When he failed to come down for his medicine at two o'clock, I decided to take it to him. Something didn't feel right and I wanted to check on him. Finding the sitting room door closed, I knocked twice and waited for his usual, "Come in."

After several seconds I knocked again. Still no answer. I could hear him in there, and it sounded as if he was moving, so he wasn't asleep. I slowly turned the knob, entered the room, and froze. Rodger was darting around the floor on all fours, pouncing like a cat chasing an elusive mouse. While I watched, he scooted across the carpet, cupping his hands to snare some invisible prey and looking under his hands to see if he'd been successful. Realizing he'd missed, he tried again and again.

I backed out of the room, closed the door, and knocked firmly three times. "Rodger, it's time for your medicine."

"Just a minute." His voice was barely audible through the door.

"Can I come in?"

"Yeah, come in."

When I entered, he was seated on the couch, his hair in disarray and his shirt pulled halfway out of his pants.

"I have your medicine."

"Thank …" He took a deep breath. "…You …" and then another breath, the recent exertion having taken its toll.

I sat beside him and waited until his breathing had settled into a normal rhythm and he'd taken his medication before handing him a glass of water and smoothing his hair away from his face.

"What's up?" he asked after taking a couple of sips and placing the glass on the table.

"Did you have a hallucination?"

"No. No hallucination. You think I see things?"

"I saw you crawling on the rug trying to catch something."

"Sometimes there's dust or string on the floor. I have to pick it up."

"No, Rodger. This wasn't dust or string. It looked like you were chasing something."

"Yeah?"

"Yes, you were moving all around the room on your hands and knees."

"Maybe I did," he said with a touch of wonder in his words. "But I don't think so," he followed up with immediately. "Sometimes a string falls on the floor and I pick it up."

"Okay," I said, knowing I'd get no further with him on that subject. "You rest for a while."

"I don't sleep much, but don't worry about me. I'm okay. You go do what you want."

I did. I went downstairs and called the doctor.

"Why do we have to go to the doctor again? In Pittsburgh, I only go every six months."

"We have to go because we need to find out why you shake like that."

His hands were trembling so hard he couldn't get his seat belt buckled, but when I reached over to help him, he pulled away.

"I can do it."

I sat back in my seat, prepared to let him try as long as he wanted. I had purposely started early to allow time for any stops I'd have to make along the way. I was disappointed when originally told it would take three weeks to get Rodger in to see the doctor again. I suspected they were sick of hearing from me and decided to wait me out. I got really mad when, on the day before I was supposed to take him in for his originally scheduled visit, I got a call saying the doctor was taking a day off and I had to reschedule.

"Can't someone else see him?"

"All the doctors are fully booked. If it's an emergency, take him in to the ER."

"When can his doctor see him?"

"We have an opening on Wednesday, two weeks from now, at 10:30 a.m."

"I'll take it."

Five weeks after seeing him chasing things across the carpet, we were on our way again. Since the initial call his behavior had become even more erratic. He paced at all hours of the day and night, sleeping only a few minutes at a time. Because of his increasing fatigue, he often lost track of time. He'd come down for breakfast in the evening, or decide it was time for his medicine an hour after taking it. Other times he'd announce he didn't need it at all and I'd have to insist he take it. He stopped shaving every other day, waiting until one of us insisted he clean himself. But, worst of all, was the shaking and ever-increasing headbobbing. I suspected Parkinson's disease. It ran in his family. His sister had it. I mentioned my suspicions to both his primary care doctor and his psychiatrist. Neither seemed to think it was the answer.

I had to call his name twice to get him restarted as we walked to the car. It stopped while he concentrated on getting his seat belt on, but returned after we were on the road for about fifteen minutes. Twice, he popped the seat belt open and reached for the door handle. I was afraid he'd forget where he was and open the door while we were moving. I struggled to keep an eye on the road and him at the same time. Each time he shifted in his seat, I'd slow down in case I had to stop fast and grab him. Cars continually passed us, some of the drivers flipping me off as they sped by. Fortunately, it was past rush hour and I wasn't causing a major traffic jam or endangering other drivers. I knew I was being a big nuisance to some people though and suspected my driving would be a topic of conversation in an office or two during the day.

"You should have seen the idiot on Route 340 this morning…"

I was relieved when Rodger started talking, just as he sometimes did in the kitchen. Every now and then, he'd use the time we had in the car to share some of his memories.

"I'm a lucky man. All my life I had food to eat, a house to live in, and a job. I did the best I could."

"Yes, you did. You worked and you raised a family and now your son can take care of you."

"I never thought I'd get married, but Shirley said she wanted to marry me. She was on welfare. She had Michael. My mother said, 'If she wants you, you should marry her. You can take care of each other.' So we get married, we have a baby, and I work in the Post Office. For the first few days, everything's nice. Then, after a couple days, she's not nice no more. Everything has to be her way. If I don't do what she says, she yells and throws a fit. I can't say nothing. I can't do nothing. Then one day she says, 'I want a divorce.'"

"Why?"

"I don't know. I said, 'You want a divorce, you get a divorce, but who will take care of the boys?' Her father said, 'You wanted to marry him. You got married. Now you want a divorce? You stay married.' So we stay married. She said, 'Who would want to marry you?' I think, 'Who would want to marry her?' She's fat. Not many men want to marry a fat woman. In the old country, they say, 'Don't marry a pretty one. An ugly girl won't cheat on you.' It was okay with me that she was fat. She was good-hearted most of time. She'd do anything for her family. Her sons, her cousins, anybody. But you couldn't tell her nothing. Everything had to be her way, that's it. I don't know why she wanted to marry me. Maybe she loved me, I don't know."

While he was talking the shaking slowed almost to a stop. I hoped he'd keep talking until we got to the hospital.

"I think she loved you," I said. "I think she had a hard time saying it, but she took good care of you. She took you to the doctor and worried about you when you were sick. You raised two fine sons together. You both did the best you could."

"I did the best I could," he agreed. "But I couldn't tell her nothing. She couldn't be different. I know I'm mentally ill. I was in the hospital for thirteen years. Always in an open ward. I did details and kept busy. Then the doctors told me I have to go home. My father is sick and my mother needs me. So I go home. Shirley was sick too, but she couldn't admit it. For a few days she took pills and everything was nice. Then she said, 'I'm not crazy, like you,' and she threw them away. I can admit I'm sick, but she couldn't. You couldn't tell her nothing. I don't know. Maybe she loved me. She married me."

An excerpt from his medical records dated April 17, 1987:

Psychological Assessment
Identifying Data: Mr. Carducci is a 60 y.o. Caucasian male who is married and unemployed.

Reason for Admission: Vet voluntarily entered HDVA on 4/16/87 at the suggestion of his wife and outpatient psychiatrist ... Vet had become more withdrawn, depressed, and disruptive at home. Wife also reported vet was behaving bizarrely (e.g., saluting her).

Psychiatric HX: Mr. Carducci reportedly suffered a psychotic break while serving in the (this section left blank in records) (1949). Records indicate symptoms at that time included confusion, auditory hallucinations, and social isolation. He was given insulin shock therapy and symptoms cleared. Adjustment thereafter was marked by lack of initiative and poverty of ideas. He was hospitalized again at the Chillicothe VH from 1950 to 1955 with subsequent transfer to the HDVA from '55 to '62. Rx consisted of ECT (20x), various meds, and structured living. Dx consistently said schizophrenia is in partial remission. Although vet was seen as capable of a higher level of functioning, he did not wish to leave the hospital. Next inpt. Stays were in '80 & '8(illegible)

Background Information: Mr. Carducci describes a deprived childhood. Father initially left the family when he was very young and family was subjected to wartime shortages. Family did eventually relocate to the U.S, yet patient did have trouble adjusting given the language and cultural barriers. This man did serve time in the military and later spent the next 12 years in the hospital. He later worked for the Post Office up until the early '80s. He has been married about 25 years and is father of two children. The marriage is marked by severe conflict, with his wife basically supervising most of his activities. Vet has threatened to divorce wife several times, yet has no strong inclination. He basically has no friends, totally relying on family for socialization.

MSE: Mr. Carducci is a short, obese man who speaks with an Italian accent. ... Most of vet's conversation consists of complaints against his wife. Speech is often irrelevant. Hygiene and grooming are poor; dress is appropriate. Movement is abrupt and swift, mostly full of jerks. Thinking is marked by slow processing, auditory hallucinations, a poverty of ideas, and rigidity. Vet would not elaborate on hallucinations he had. ... Vet was somewhat preoccupied with fantasies about having "another wife and a better life." Associations were logical and fairly well organized; cognitive processing was fairly simple & concrete. Intelligence is estimated to be below average. Some actions taken by vet are immature, inappropriate, and bizarre. Vet described some actions he does at home (e.g., setting clocks wrong & barking at wife to get back at her for "controlling him"); mood was moderately to severely depressed. Though vet complained of irritability and at times rage at his wife, underlying effect is anger, which is inappropriate. Action is chronically low, as is energy. Eating is excessive, whereas sleeping varies greatly. At times of depression sleep is quite low. Presently sleep is averaging 6 hr. nightly. Suicidal notions are denied though vet wishes to be dead. Homicidal notions are likewise denied. Insight and judgment are nil. Impulse control is fair. Alcohol & substance abuse are denied. Social isolation is chronic.

Conclusions: pt impresses as

I: Schizoaffective Disorder

II: Deferred

III. s/p bilateral cataract surgery

Negative symptoms of schizophrenia, as well as depressed mood, most notable. Flo?? Psychosis is not seen. Marital conflict is severe, and vet appears to be deliberately engaging in some inappropriate behavior to "get back at wife." Recommend time-out period for family & vet's sake, med stabilization, and encouragement to express feelings in a more mature way.

I wondered when I read the last few words of that evaluation, "encouragement to express feelings in a more mature way," if the doctor had any idea how impossible that would've been. Not only was my father-in-law incapable of the type of introspection that would allow him to express his feelings, my mother-in-law wouldn't have listened. She was a volatile woman who insisted everything be done her way. She'd start out using persuasion to get what she wanted, but if that didn't work she'd resort to passive aggressive behavior that would make changing the time on a clock, or barking at your spouse, look like child's play. Rodger couldn't speak up to her. Mike was one of very few people who ever could, and even he said the best thing he did for our marriage was move four hours away from his mother.

On the surface it would appear that they were bad for one another, but in an odd way they were uniquely suited. She was a single mother at a time when single mothers were rare. She wanted to get off welfare and build a better life for herself and her son. She wasn't a pretty woman, and she struggled all her life with her weight, but she did have a good heart. She took care of her family. He was a mentally ill, disabled veteran who probably would've deteriorated without a family to care for. Together, they got her off the welfare rolls, bought a home, and raised their children. They were married almost forty years. I hope she loved him.

I breathed a long sigh of relief when we finally arrived at the gate to the hospital.

"What brings you back so soon?" the doctor asked.

"It's not really so soon," I reminded him. While it was true I had called soon after his last appointment, it had taken well over a month to get in to see him.

"You're right," he admitted, looking at Rodger's chart. "What's going on?"

"The day I called, I had just walked into his room and found him crawling on the floor chasing something that wasn't there. When I asked him if he was having hallucinations, he said no. But when I described what he'd been doing, he said, 'Hmm, maybe I did.'

"Sometimes I hear him laughing hysterically in his room. He's all alone in there, Doctor. He's talking and he's laughing and he's shaking and spinning."

"Spinning?"

"Yes. He lifts his arms and raises one leg and spins like a ballerina or a skater. Often when we come out of our bedroom, he's standing just outside the door. Then he runs down the hall into his bedroom, convinced he fooled us into thinking he was there all along. But the worst thing to watch is the headbanging. It has to hurt. I'm afraid he'll end up with a brain injury it's so forceful sometimes. The hand tremors are increasing too."

"I hesitate to increase his medication again," the doctor warned. "He's on a high dose now, and there are serious side effects to these drugs. What do you want me to do?"

I wanted to respond with, "I want you to tell me what's going on. I want you to put him back the way he was when he came to live with us last year." But I'd said that so many times in the past months I knew it wouldn't get me anywhere.

"I don't have an answer to that, Doctor. That's why I keep bringing him back. You have to tell me what options we have for finding out what this is."

"Let's rule out Parkinson's disease," he said. "You mentioned there's a family history of it, isn't that right?"

"Yes, his sister had it. What do we have to do to get him tested?"

"I'll put in for a consult with a neurologist, and the office will call you to set up an appointment."

"When?"

"That depends on when there's an opening."

"Can you mark it urgent?"

"I'll make a note that you want him to be seen as soon as possible. Are you having hallucinations, Mr. Carducci?"

"No. She worries about me." He chuckled. "I tell her I'm fine. When you get old, you shake. She shouldn't bother you. I just don't sleep much."

The two of them repeated the same series of questions and answers that were always a part of a psych visit, questions about his feeling suicidal or homicidal, or if he was depressed or not. These questions had been asked and answered so many times over the years Rodger knew they were coming and knew what the right answers should be. I wondered why doctors took the word of a sick person, one who has had multiple admissions to psychiatric hospitals, over that of his caregivers. He'd had at least one hallucination. I'd seen it. Who knew how many more had occurred during the hours he was alone in his room.

Rodger shook and twitched and headbanged the whole way to the hospital the afternoon of his appointment with the neurologist. I tried talking to him, hoping to keep him focused and alleviate some of his symptoms. He was really out of it, and I was very frightened.

Please don't jump out of this car, I prayed.

"He doesn't have Parkinson's disease," the neurologist stated firmly. "In fact, I see no sign of any type of neurological problems in your father."

"Father-in-law," I corrected him.

It irritated me that people at the hospital couldn't seem to get our relationship right, despite the fact that his records say exactly who I am. How much of his chart do they actually read?

"In any case," the doctor continued, "there's nothing I can do for him. I haven't seen him manifest any of the symptoms you describe."

It was true. As soon as we entered the doctor's office, Rodger had stopped twitching.

How does he do this? How can he be so out of control at home and in the car and then sit here and calmly fake out the doctor?

"Doctor, if you walk down the hall with me and wait for five minutes, I guarantee that when we come back in this room he'll be shaking his head in some kind of seizure."

"That may be true," he answered, his tone clearly skeptical, "but I have another patient to see, and as I've already said, I haven't seen any involuntary movements from him."

"It happens all the time. What do I have to do to convince you? Videotape him?"

"That's an excellent idea," he answered, ushering us toward the door. "Why don't you do that, and if you're able to capture these tremors on tape, bring it to me and I'll take a look."

As soon as we got into the car he started headbanging and shaking again. He struggled to put his seat belt on but refused to let me help him.

"You can go," he said. "I'll get it."

"I'm not moving the car until it's on."

"There," he said after several tries.

He was lying.

"No. It's not hooked and I know it."

"Just go. You don't need it all the time."

"Yes you do. Let me help you."

"No, I can do it."

"Then do it. I'm in no hurry. I'll wait as long as it takes."

After several minutes of near misses and exasperated sighs, I heard the telltale click I'd been waiting for and started the car.

I knew he wasn't happy with me; every now and then he'd look over and mutter something under his breath. I ignored his little fit of temper and concentrated on driving.

Then I heard it. He'd unhooked the belt.

"Put that back on," I told him.

"I don't need it," he insisted.

"Yes you do. It's the law. Put it back on." I slowed the car, looking for a safe place to pull over.

"Why'd you stop?" he asked when I turned off the engine.

"I can't drive until you're safe. You have to wear your belt."

I was more afraid that he'd open the door and jump out than I was of getting into an accident, but I couldn't tell him that. Fortunately, I had the law on my side and could use that as my reason to make him wear it.

With a little less trouble than he'd had the first time, he snapped the belt into place and I started the car. We'd only gone about five miles when I heard him snap it open again.

I didn't say a word. I just slowed the car and pulled off on the side again. This time, I put the keys in my purse and held it securely on my lap.

"Aren't you going to go?" he asked after several moments of silence had passed.

"I can't."

"Why not?"

"You have to put on your belt."

"It's too tight."

"I'm sorry if that's true, but you still have to wear it."

"Not all the time."

"All the time when the car is moving."

That time he waited ten minutes before putting it on. As soon as it was in place, I started the car and pulled onto the road again.

We had only gone a few hundred yards when he took it off again. Again I pulled over to the side of the road and stopped the engine. And waited … And waited … And waited.

"You better drive," he said. "It's going to take a long time to get home if you keep stopping."

"I don't mind. I'll wait all night if I have to. I can't drive until you put on your seatbelt."

"No."

"Okay, we'll just sit here all night."

Watching me put the key in the ignition a few minutes later, he must have thought I'd given in. He looked at me with a grin of satisfaction and crossed his arms, as if to say, "I showed you, didn't I?"

That look of triumph disappeared and he tilted his head and lowered one eyebrow in an expression of confusion when, instead of starting the car, I turned on the radio and started singing. Loud singing. Out-of-tune singing. Really bad singing. I wasn't deliberately trying to sing badly; I can't help it. I often wish I could sing, but since I can't I decided to use my lack of talent to my best advantage. When the first song ended, I caught him looking over at me, probably hoping I'd give up and drive on. He was out of luck. As soon as another song started, I did too. Even if I didn't know the words, I kept on singing with the radio.

Finally, he couldn't take it anymore.

"Stop ... singing...," he demanded through clenched teeth.

"Not until you put on your seatbelt," I countered, my teeth clenched as tightly as his.

He gave up. And as soon as he had the belt on, I turned the radio off and started the car. The seatbelt stayed on the rest of the way home.

We were about halfway there when he looked over at me and said, "You're a little bit crazy, I think."

"Yep, but I sure can sing, can't I?" I grinned.

He just shook his head and sighed.

That evening, Mike put the video camera on a tripod and set it up in the family room. It was in plain sight; we had no desire to hide anything from Rodger or anyone else.

When he was upstairs, we pointed the camera toward the hall between his rooms. When he was downstairs, we aimed it toward the kitchen. Within a day or two it was just another piece of furniture. Some of the things we saw when we played back that tape were deeply disturbing. Unfortunately, by the time his doctor got around to playing the tape it was too late to do any good.

One afternoon shortly after it was installed, I came in from a quick run to the store and went upstairs to put my shoes away. I was almost to the top when I sensed movement low and off to the right. Rodger was on all fours again, only this time he wasn't chasing anything. His movements were slow and deliberate. He'd raise one hand like a lion's paw then hesitate and look around before placing it on the floor. Then he'd raise the opposite hand and do the same thing. I watched him go to the end of the hall, nudge open the door to my bedroom with his head, and peer in.

"What are you looking for?" I asked him, hoping to bring him out of it as I had the first time I saw him hallucinating.

Upon hearing my voice, he turned quickly and started crawling toward me, moving faster than I thought possible.

He's coming after me! My heart started racing as fear swept over me. Thoughts of how to escape raced through my mind. Time seemed to stand still as panic continued to build—until he suddenly stopped advancing. Whatever he was seeing, it wasn't me. At that moment, he was somewhere far away, startled and crazed with hatred for something only he could see. *I pray I can outrun him!* I thought, visualizing an impending attack. Under normal conditions there would be no doubt, but who knew what he was capable of in that state.

"Rodger, wake up," I ordered, hoping my voice sounded a lot more confident than I felt. "Get up off the floor and go to your room."

Thank God, he obeyed.

"What were you doing?"

"I thought I heard a noise, that's all. I'm tired now."

Me too, I thought as my heart rate slowed to normal. I was exhausted from the strain of the past few minutes, and relieved I'd been able to bring him out of his trance. The next day all hell broke loose.

Chapter 6

Rodger paced all morning. When he wasn't pacing, he was headbobbing and headbanging more than ever.

"Is this food any good?" he asked when I put lunch on the table.

"The food is fine," I reassured him again.

A week before, a hurricane had knocked the power out for three days. He'd asked that same question every day since the storm came through. Not willing to take any chances with his health, or ours, Mike had thrown out anything that might have gone bad and replaced it as soon as the power was back on.

"Remember, I told you this morning that we got new food after the storm?"

"I hope it's all right," he answered, sniffing his plate.

"Do you want something else?"

"No. I'll eat it. I hope it's good."

He ate it, but he put each forkful up to his nose and gave it a good long sniff before putting it into his mouth. I wondered how long it would take to convince him that the food was fresh and safe to eat.

When he finished and tried to put his plate into the dishwasher, he got stuck in place three times trying to walk across the kitchen. Once there, he froze and shook his head violently. It took several tries to bring him out of it.

"Why don't you go and lie down for a while," I suggested. "Maybe after a nap you'll feel better."

"When does he see the doctor again?" Mike asked. "He's worse than ever today."

"I know. I'm going to call again in the morning. If I can't get him in to see the neurologist, I'll take him to the emergency room and I'll sit there until someone pays attention to this."

Mike nodded in agreement and then pointed toward the stairs. His dad was coming down again.

"I want to talk to my brother."

Rodger's brother lived about forty minutes away, but the two rarely saw one another. There was an awkwardness between them that was difficult to understand. Still, they maintained a bond that was important to Rodger. Mike and I encouraged visits and readily dialed the phone when Rodger wanted to talk to him.

"Here you go." Mike quickly punched in the numbers and handed the phone to his father.

From what we could hear, the call was typical of the two.

"Hi. How are you doing? How's the family? Say hello to everybody. Goodbye."

Rodger handed the phone to Mike and went back upstairs. When he didn't come down at 2:00 for his medicine, Mike took it up to him. When he opened the door, the sound of his father's laughter spilled out.

"What was so funny?" I asked when Mike came back down.

"Hell if I know. He was standing in the middle of the room laughing his ass off about something. When I asked what was so funny, he just took the medicine and sat down. He wouldn't even look at me."

"This is getting too freaking weird. He is definitely going to the hospital tomorrow."

Things remained quiet for the rest of the afternoon. After a while Mike went out to do some yard work, and I got busy with some light housekeeping and started making preparations for the evening meal.

"Rodger, dinner's ready," I called.

He'd been up from his nap for a while. I could hear him pacing, heavy-footed, down the hall and back. Each time he reached the point just outside the bathroom, I'd hear the floor squeak. Then he'd mutter something incomprehensible. *Pace, pace, pace, pace, squeak, mutter. Pace, pace, pace, pace, squeak, mutter.* He was stuck in motion. Again. Tears of frustration welled in my eyes and I prayed someone would be able to figure this out soon.

"Rodger, are you hungry?" I called again.

"No," he shouted back. "I'm not eating anything you cook anymore."

"What? Why?"

"No more food! No more food from you! I know what you're trying to do!"

"Dad, what's the matter?" Mike called to him.

By then he was running back and forth along the hallway, agitated and shaking the banister as he went.

"You're trying to poison me. I know it!"

"You think we want to hurt you?" Mike demanded.

"No food. I'm not taking anything from her again! She puts poison in it. I've seen her. I know what she's up to. I want the phone. I'm calling the police."

Mike and I looked at each other. In little more than a glance we communicated shock, dismay, and confusion.

"You want to call the police?! Mike shouted.

"Yes. I don't trust you. I don't trust her. No more of your tricks. No more. Call the cops."

"Fine," Mike snapped. "You want the police, we'll call the police."

"What are you saying?" I asked him. "He's sick. We have to get him to the hospital. Don't holler at him."

"I'm trying to show him we'll go along and call the cops," he explained.

I looked up the stairs and saw my father-in-law, wild-eyed and frantic. His scary, unreadable stare sent a chill down my spine.

Mike had just come down from taking a shower before dinner.

"Go get your shoes," I told him. "We have to take him to the hospital."

As he headed for the stairs, I turned back to the stove, shutting off the burners one by one. I looked at the large cook's knife I'd used to chop the vegetables for dinner.

Hide it, a little voice inside me whispered. *Don't let him see it.*

I felt an instant rush of guilt and shame for even thinking such a thing, but his behavior was so erratic I didn't dare take any chances.

Don't overreact. He's sick but he's not dangerous.

And then I heard his footsteps on the stairs.

Quickly, I scooped up the razor-sharp knife, wrapped the blade in a thick kitchen towel, and stuffed it into the nearest drawer, putting my body between the cabinet and anyone coming near.

I needn't have worried; he didn't even glance in my direction. Upon reaching the bottom of the stairs, he rushed down the entrance hall and out the front door, muttering under his breath as he went.

"I have to get out. Can't trust her. Can't trust him. Call the cops."

"Mike, he's taken off!" I yelled, running for the door, hoping Mike had heard me, but not waiting for a response.

I can't believe he can move this fast, was the first thing that ran through my mind as I increased my speed, trying to catch him before he got too far. I was in excellent shape for a woman my age, due to years of regular aerobic exercise and weight training, but it was clear it was going to be tough to catch him. Between the head start he'd gotten and the demons driving him, he was increasing the distance between us with each step.

God, don't let him drop over from a heart attack before I catch him. You better hope he runs out of gas before you get too far yourself, my damned inner voice chided, reminding me that no matter how fit I thought I was, it had been a long time since I'd run a 5K—and I'd never been a sprinter.

Still, he's a sick old man. He's over seventy, for Pete's sake.

I had no sooner completed that thought than he veered to the right and headed up the driveway of a nearby home.

"Thanks for listening, Lord," I said out loud, gladly slowing my pace when I realized where he'd gone for help.

It had been a comfort seeing the distinctive brown sheriff's car parked in the driveway just a few doors down each night. The selling agent had bragged that there were several members of the clergy and many law enforcement officers living in the development, along with a mix of professionals and growing families that would keep enrollment steady in the nearby elementary school for many years to come. I was relieved to see that even through the haze of mental illness clouding his mind, Rodger was still lucid enough to remember where to find a safe haven.

"Stay away from me!" he shouted, frantically pushing on the doorbell. "Get away. I know what you're trying to do. I need to go to the hospital. It's safe there. They have to take me. They have to take me, they promised."

"Rodger, listen to me. It's okay. Come back to the house and Mike will take you to the hospital."

"No! Can't trust him. Can't trust you. I'm calling the cops."

The couple in the next house was busy unloading groceries from their car, their arms full of bags, when they noticed the commotion.

"He's sick," I told them. "I'm trying to get him to go to the hospital but he's afraid of me. He's my father-in-law, and he lives with us right down the street."

I looked over my shoulder for Mike but there was no sign of him. I knew then that he hadn't heard me call out to him and I was on my own.

Just then the door opened and a man stepped out.

"Help me," Rodger cried. "You gotta help me. I can't trust them. She poisons me all the time. I know it. I gotta go to the hospital. Can't trust her."

"He's sick," I told the off-duty deputy sheriff. "We live two doors over. He's delusional. I need help to get him to go with me."

"No, don't listen," Rodger interrupted. "Help me."

"Believe me, officer," I pleaded. "He's paranoid. We were getting ready to take him to the hospital when he suddenly ran out of the house and came here."

"Look, lady," the deputy spoke up. "This is my home and this is my day off. Get him off my property or I'll arrest both of you."

"No, you don't understand," Rodger pleaded. "I can't trust her.

I have to go to the hospital. She tries to poison me."

"Get him out of here." the deputy repeated. "I don't appreciate your bringing him to my home like this. Both of you get out of here right now."

"I didn't bring him here," I tried to explain, not only to him but to the neighbors who were now listening as well. "He ran out of the house. I was afraid he'd get lost or hurt so I followed him. My husband and I were getting ready to take him to the hospital when he took off."

"Where do you live?" the deputy demanded.

"Two doors down." I pointed.

"Do as I say and get him out of here."

"No, I can't go with her." Rodger pleaded, sweat pouring off him and carrying the smell of fear across the lawn. He reached out to the deputy.

"Back away, now." the cop demanded. Looking away from Rodger and toward me, he said, "I'm warning you one more time. Either you both get off my property right now, or I'm going to call another sheriff's car and have you both arrested."

I looked toward the people next door for help but they were gone. I looked back toward home and still there was no sign of Mike. I was desperate for help.

"Do it," I said.

"What?"

"Call for another car and have us arrested. If that's the only way I can get help for him, do it."

From the look on his face I knew he hadn't expected that response, but before he had a chance to say anything, Rodger started pleading with him again.

"Help me. You gotta help me. She's poisoning me."

"No, sir, I don't have to help you. Get off my property or I'm going to arrest you. Do you hear me?"

"You're a cop aren't you?"

"Yes, I'm a deputy sheriff, and if you don't leave now you will be arrested."

"But you're a cop and I need help."

"I don't care." he stated firmly.

"You're a cop and you don't care? You have to care." A confused look crossed Rodger's face as he tried to process this information.

"No. I don't care," the deputy insisted. "I don't care about you, and I don't care what your problems are. Just get out of here."

The deputy looked back toward me. "Can't you get him out of here? If you don't, you're both going to jail. You say he lives with you. Can't you control him?"

"Not now I can't. He thinks I'm trying to hurt him. If I come close I don't know what he'll do."

"Where do you live?" he demanded again.

"Right over there," I told him, pointing once more.

"Who else lives there?"

"My husband. This man's son. He went to get his shoes so we could take his dad to the hospital when he ran out and came here."

"Go get him." he demanded.

With a quick look at my father-in-law, I took off running, hoping he would still be there when I got back.

I opened the front door just in time to see Mike come down the staircase. "Hurry up. Your father ran away. He's down at the deputy's house telling him we're trying to kill him."

"That's good," Mike replied. "He can help us get him calmed down."

"No he won't." I tried to explain and get him moving faster. "He ordered us off his property and is threatening to arrest Rodger and me if we don't stop bothering him."

"What???"

"Come on," I urged. "Hurry up. This guy is no help at all. He's mad at us for disturbing his day off, and he's going to call another car and have us taken in."

"Let him try," Mike snorted.

"Hell, I told him to do it. I figure if that's the only way to get help, I'll go for a ride in a sheriff's car."

"I'm sure it won't come to that," my husband reasoned. "I'll talk to him."

"You can try. I sure hope he listens to you better than he listens to me."

When Mike and I arrived at his house, the deputy was coming out the front door. Rodger was still begging him for help and getting nowhere.

"Are these people related to you?" the deputy demanded of Mike.

"Yes, sir. This is my wife, Bobbi, and this is my father, Rodger. My father is sick and we need your help."

"I already told her and now I'm telling you. Get him off my property or he'll be arrested and so will you."

"My wife told you he's sick and needs to go to the hospital. Is that right?"

"Yes. She told me. And I told her I don't care what your problems are. I'm not going to help you on my day off."

"I don't believe this," Mike said.

Suddenly I remembered something. "Go get the other cop, the one that lives on the next block."

While my worried husband took off between the houses in search of help, the angry deputy went into his house and slammed the door, leaving me standing watch over Rodger, wondering if I was about to spend the night in jail.

Chapter 7

Rodger and I locked eyes across the yard. The scent of warm grass and fear mixed in the early evening air. *His fear or mine?* I wondered, admitting that I was as afraid of him as he was of me at that moment. I'd heard that crazy people have tremendous strength, and I didn't doubt he'd use every ounce of it to defend himself if I got too close.

"Stay back," he shouted, starting to pace again. "I know. They think I don't but I do. Bastards are trying to kill me."

"Rodger, it's me. It's Bobbi. I won't hurt you."

"You lie," he whimpered. "I have to go. Have to run. He doesn't care." He glanced at the house. "A man against humanity. It don't make sense. I have to go."

"Don't move," I pleaded. "Mike went to get help. I won't hurt you, I promise. Just wait a minute. Help is coming." I tried to use a soothing tone but even I could hear the panic in my voice.

"No more waiting." His voice trembled. "Can't trust." He picked up his pace, back and forth across the lawn. This time I was grateful to discover he was stuck in a pattern of movement that could last for several minutes, provided no one spoke.

C'mon Mike, I prayed, looking around and hoping to spot him coming with reinforcements before his father came out of his latest spell and decided to take off again.

Rodger must have heard them before I did. He suddenly cocked his head and started to move toward the side of the house. I braced myself and took in a deep breath, preparing to start running again, when Mike came around the corner, followed by a sheriff and the two neighbors I thought had abandoned me.

"Thank you," I mouthed to the woman as she passed on the way to her home.

She acknowledged my gratitude with a nod of her head and a whispered, "Good luck," before disappearing into her house.

The new man on the scene approached Rodger with caution,

introducing himself in a soft and reassuring tone of voice. "Mr. Carducci, I'm Sheriff Green. I understand you need some help. What can I do for you, sir?"

"Call the cops. I need the cops. I can't trust them no more."

"I'm with the sheriff's office, Mr. Carducci. I'll help you. Can you calm down and tell me what the problem is?"

"I need to go to the hospital. They have to take me. She's trying to poison me. I can't stay here. Don't let them touch me."

The wild look in his eyes intensified each time he glanced at me. I kept expecting him to lunge, wondering what they could do if that happened. Despite his irrational behavior, regardless of the fear his illness touched off in me, he was still an old man with brittle bones and an artificial valve in his heart. Restraining him would only increase his paranoia. Allowing him to run could result in a heart attack.

"Try to calm yourself, Mr. Carducci," the sheriff reassured him. "I'll do everything I can to help you. I won't let anyone hurt you. What do you want to do?"

"Call the hospital."

"Do you want me to call the hospital?"

"No. I call the hospital. Can't trust nobody."

"All right, Mr. Carducci, you can call the hospital. You can use my phone." He extended his arm toward Rodger, offering his cell phone. "Do you have the number?"

"No. She has it. I can't trust her," he whimpered.

"Can you get me the number?" the sheriff asked.

I nodded and took off to the house to get it.

I don't know what happened while I was gone, maybe it was just my leaving that reassured him, but by the time I got back with the number for the hospital, Rodger was much calmer. I quickly passed the number to the sheriff and stepped back. He dialed and handed the phone to Rodger, stepping away to allow him to speak freely.

While Rodger was on the phone with the hospital, the deputy

came out of his house and spoke to the other officer.

"I've already called a car to take care of this," he told him. "They should be here any minute. I told them repeatedly to vacate my property and they refused."

I couldn't hear what was said between them, but the next thing I knew, the first one had a new attitude and Sheriff Green was speaking into his radio.

"Mike Green here. I understand you have a car on the way to Magic Mountain Drive in Round Hill. Yes. Yes … We have a confused elderly man requesting assistance. I'm working with the family to get him to a hospital for treatment. No. No need for that … She didn't do anything wrong. No. No one is in trouble here. Go ahead and send a car to transport Mr. Carducci to the hospital where he can be assessed for treatment."

Ending the call, he turned back to Rodger. "How's it going, sir?"

"They can't come and get me. I can't trust anyone. I need to go to the hospital."

"I'll see to it you get to the hospital. A car will be here soon to take you to the nearest hospital. They'll help you."

Soon the car arrived and two more deputies stepped out. The female went directly to Rodger, offering to take him into our house to retrieve anything he wanted to take with him.

Recognizing that others were taking a different view of the situation, the first deputy approached in an attempt to appear supportive.

"He'll be at the hospital soon. I'm sure he'll be fine," he said, nodding toward Rodger, who was now sitting in the back seat of the sheriff's car, preparing for the drive to the hospital.

"Get away from me." I snapped. "Your behavior has been the most unprofessional display of insensitivity to a man in trouble I have ever seen."

Startled by my reaction, he stepped closer to Mike and attempted to speak with him.

"I'd hate to think what might have happened if my father had been in the hands of someone who wanted to harm him." Mike glared at the man. "He was pleading for help and you ordered him off your lawn because it's your day off. What the hell is wrong with you?"

I couldn't understand it. How could anyone, let alone a neighbor and a member of the sheriff's department, react with such callous disregard for an old man asking for help?

I decided that once things calmed down, I'd tell everyone in the neighborhood what he had done, and lodge an official complaint with the sheriff's office. After thanking everyone who had come to our aid, Mike and I got into our car and drove to the local hospital to find out what would happen next.

Rodger was still highly agitated when we got there. Unable to communicate his needs to the doctor in the ER, other than to repeat his accusations against his family and to plead for help, he was pacing, headbanging, and mumbling, refusing to allow anyone to touch him. The doctor listened carefully to our explanation about how Rodger had ended up arriving at the hospital in a police car, and gratefully accepted the list of his medications I had grabbed before leaving the house.

"Mr. Carducci, stop that," the doctor ordered when Rodger had a particularly violent episode of headshaking.

"I can't stop," he answered. "She makes me do it. She tries to control me with food."

After reviewing his list of meds and hearing that Rodger was a patient at the VA hospital, it was decided that the best thing to do was get him medicated and calm and take him there where he'd be admitted into the care of doctors familiar with his case.

"Will you let your son and daughter-in-law drive you to the hospital, Mr. Carducci?" the doctor asked once the tranquilizer began to take hold.

"No. I can't trust. You take me."

"I can't do that, sir. I have to stay here and take care of sick people. Will you let them take you?"

"No. I'll stay here."

"You can't stay here. I'll tell you what. It should take you less than hour to get there. You go with your son and daughter-in-law, and I'll call the hospital and tell them you're on the way. If you don't arrive safely within an hour, they'll call the police and tell them to arrest your son and his wife. Can you do that, sir?"

"I can't stay here?"

"No. You need to be with your own doctors."

"Okay, but I don't want them to sit by me. I can't trust."

"I'll tell them to sit in the front seat. You stay in the back. They won't be able to reach you. Are you ready to go?"

"If I have to."

"It's for the best," the doctor reassured him.

No one spoke on the drive to the hospital. Mike and I were lost in our own thoughts, trying to process what had just happened. As the sun set and darkness descended into the car, I could hear Rodger mumbling and moving in the back seat. The smell of fear still lingered in the air. His breathing sounded like a panting dog on the prowl.

I felt tremendous guilt for thinking that way. I didn't want to spook him by continually looking back at him, but I remained alert to his presence, hoping he didn't decide to loop a seat belt around my neck as we drove through the mountains.

When we were almost there, Mike turned to me. "Are you okay?"

"I'm okay," I reassured him, not convincing either one of us. "He's sick and he needs treatment. This is the best thing for him right now."

Reluctantly, Mike agreed while pretending he was fine too. The truth is, we were deeply shaken by what we'd just witnessed.

Rodger almost ran into the emergency room when we arrived at the hospital. He went directly to the check-in office and informed the attendant that he was being poisoned and demanded to be admitted.

"He's a psych patient and he's having a breakdown. He called here earlier trying to get someone to pick him up and bring him in. He thinks I'm trying to hurt him."

"Who are you?" the man asked.

"I'm his daughter-in-law. He lives with his son and me. We have his medical power of attorney so you can talk to either one or both of us."

"Mr. Carducci," a nurse spoke upon entering the room. "I'm glad you got here." She turned to me. "He called us. We couldn't understand half of what he said, and we didn't know if you were aware he was calling or not."

I filled her in on what had happened and then she took Rodger back into an examining room to be assessed. Mike joined me a few minutes later, having gone to park the car.

Within an hour Rodger had been admitted to the psychiatric ward. We were told to call in the morning to speak to the floor nurse and to expect a call from his doctor later in the day.

"Thank God you can take me," Rodger told the nurse as he was led away. "They're trying to kill me. She poisons the food. I can't trust nobody. Is the food any good here?"

The news from the doctor the following afternoon was not good.

"He's very angry with you both, and he's highly delusional. It would be best if you stay away for a few days. He's hearing voices and exhibiting some posturing that concerns me."

"Do you have an idea how long he'll need to be there?" Mike asked.

"It's too soon to guess, but I'd plan on at least two to three weeks. It takes a while for the medication to work and getting the right dose often takes some doing as well. We'll keep you updated on his progress. Exactly how long had he been acting out before you decided to bring him in?"

I didn't care for the tone of that last question. It was a good thing that Mike answered before I did.

"Which time?" Mike asked.

Clearly puzzled, the doctor asked, "What do you mean, which time? I don't see any notes about a previous psychiatric admission."

"You wouldn't, because there hasn't been one. We tried for months to find out what was wrong with my father. Check his medical and his psychiatric outpatient visits and you'll see that my wife has been seeking answers for his behavior for a long time."

"That's good." The doctor cleared his throat, his tone less critical this time. "I'm glad to hear he's with people who care."

"He certainly is," Mike assured him, "and we'll stay away as you suggest, for his sake. But one of us will be calling every day for an update."

And we did. The house seemed empty without Rodger, and several times I caught myself listening for the sound of pacing or looking to see if he was peering down at me from the upstairs hall. We knew he was extremely sick and it would take time for him to recover, but we were totally unprepared for what we heard six weeks later.

After several attempts at finding the right medication at the right dose, the doctor advised us to be prepared to commit him to a long-term care facility.

"He's not responding to treatment. He may never be able to live outside a hospital again."

Mike and I were deeply shaken. He'd been hospitalized many times before and he'd always bounced back.

"Is there nothing more to be done?" Mike asked.

"We'll keep trying, but I'm not as hopeful as I was at the time he was admitted. I recommend commitment to the psychiatric ward at Perry Point. It won't happen overnight, and while we wait for transfer we'll continue to treat him. We haven't tried electroconvulsive therapy yet. There's a slight chance that will work."

We wouldn't hear of it. Despite the fact that ECT today is much different than it was in the 1960s, we couldn't put him through that.

Rodger told us many times about the last time it was done to him.

"I knew they were coming to do electric shock. I tried and tried to resist but it was no use. I was going to fight until I died but they were too strong. They tied me up in a straitjacket and I had to give up. I couldn't fight no more. They did it even when I didn't want it. I don't know why. After that they didn't do it anymore and I don't know why not. They just do what they want. They don't care what you say."

"Ice baths were not too bad," he'd told me. "Once you get as cold as you can get, it makes you relax, but electric shock is no good. One time they wanted my mother to sign for experimental treatment. They wanted to put a needle in the back of my brain. My mother said no. Three other men, their families said yes. They all died. My mother saved my life."

The last thing we wanted was to have him locked up in a mental hospital for the rest of his life, but we knew he'd rather die than undergo electric shock again. We tried to prepare ourselves for the move.

"Mrs. Carducci?" an unfamiliar voice on the phone inquired.

"Yes, who is this?"

"My name is John and I'm calling from the VA hospital. Your father has been discharged and I need to know what time you can come and get him."

"He's going to be discharged? When?"

"Today. How long will it take you to get here?"

I didn't know what to think. Did he have the wrong number? Was this a joke?

"Are you calling about Rodger Carducci?"

"Yes. When can I expect you?"

"I'm not sure." My thoughts were reeling from the sudden change in plan.

"I need to know," the man insisted.

"And I need to know what's going on. We were told he was to be transferred to a long-term care facility. That he was too sick to ever come home."

"Who told you that?"

"His doctor."

"His doctor signed the release this morning. When can you get here?"

"I don't know. I'll have to call you back."

I needed time to think, and I needed to call Mike and tell him about this. Something was wrong, and I had the feeling it was going to take both of us find out what it was.

"I must hear from you soon. He has to be out of here tonight."

"I said I'll call you back. Give me your extension number."

Mike was as confused as I was when I reached him. He took the man's name and number and told me to sit tight. He'd find out what was going on and call me back.

"I was told the same thing you were," Mike reported a few minutes later. "And when I pushed to find out how this could happen so fast when we'd been told he was never coming home, I was informed that they tried to get him admitted to long-term care and there was no room for him. When I protested that this was outrageous, the man I was speaking with changed his tune, said that the medicine was working, Dad was well enough to come home, and it had to be today."

"What do we do now?"

"We go to the hospital and talk to this guy face to face."

When we arrived we were ushered into a room with two people we'd never seen before: a social worker and a representative from the Mental Health Intensive Case Management (MHICM) Program. They explained that the nurse would work closely with us to monitor Rodger at home. He'd do weekly home visits to make sure he was taking his medication and do all he could to help us keep Rodger out of the hospital in the future.

"Don't worry. I won't be coming into your home and taking over. I'll be there to support you."

"There's no way I'd allow you to come into my home and take over anything," I assured him, using the same imperious tone he used when speaking to us. "I don't know you. I have no idea what this program is, and I want to know who made these decisions without talking to us."

"What's the problem?" the other man asked. "Don't you want your father back?"

I could see from the look on his face that Mike was getting as angry as I was. We had never done anything to indicate we didn't want his father back. We did want answers as to how and why this quick change in plan came about. The question was never answered to our satisfaction. After a while Rodger was led into the room. He'd lost twenty-five pounds since his admission and his clothes hung on him. He appeared to be half asleep, but he smiled when he saw us.

"Mr. Carducci," the social worker spoke, "your family is here to take you home. Are you ready to go?"

"No," he answered quietly, looking at his feet.

It was clear from the surprised look on his face that the social worker hadn't expected him to say that.

"I'll stay here. I don't mind."

"You can't stay here, Mr. Carducci. It's time to go home."

Rodger didn't respond.

"Is there something wrong at home? Are they mean to you?"

"No, everything's nice." He sounded breathless and he coughed every few minutes.

"Do you have a cold?" I asked him.

"No, everything's nice."

"Mr. Carducci, it's time to go home," he was told again.

"I can stay here. I'm used to living in a hospital."

The social worker ignored him, and after a few more minutes of talk that got us no closer to an answer about how or why we were summoned that day, we took Rodger home.

In what I thought was an effort to placate us, the social worker walked with us to the door and said, "We are always here for him if he needs us. Take him home, and if you end up having to bring him back, do it."

Rodger sat quietly in the back seat, far more subdued than on the day we'd taken him in. The only sound was his almost-constant cough.

When we got home, we helped him directly to his room and put him to bed. The insistent cough went on throughout the night and all the next day. When he tried to eat the cough would get worse; it was the same when he drank anything. He was very tired and it was a chore for him to go up and down the stairs. When I woke to the sound of an incessant cough the following morning, I knew he had to go back to the hospital. I thought of the social worker's parting words, convinced he knew when we left that it wouldn't be for long.

As soon as we arrived at the emergency room, he was ushered into a room and a blood oxygen monitor was placed on his finger. The reading was dangerously low and he was put on oxygen right away.

"We're back," I greeted the nurse.

"Well, you shouldn't be," she snapped. "I know you don't want to take care of him at home, but this is no place for a sick person. Hospitals are full of germs, and if he gets an infection he could die. You aren't doing him any favors by bringing him here."

"You tell me," I snapped back at her, "how I can take care of him at home when he's this sick. He can't breathe, he's barely conscious, and he can't eat or drink anything."

I was so angry I didn't trust myself to speak anymore, and Mike was also at the boiling point.

"Forget it." The nurse backed off.

I kept my mouth shut but I had no intention of forgetting any of this. First, I'd get him the care he needed ,and then I'd deal with how we ended up at the hospital again.

It was another Sunday when he was readmitted to the hospital; the doctor of record wouldn't be in until morning. We were told

Rodger would be carefully monitored through the night, and the doctor would call us in the morning.

"You're father has pneumonia," we were informed the next day. "He's very sick, and he'll need to stay here for a week to ten days."

Later that evening the doctor called, telling us that Rodger was being moved to the Intensive Care Unit as a precaution.

"Due to his age and his medical history, we think it would be better for him to be monitored more closely than can be done on the general ward. There's no reason to be alarmed. He's getting the best care available."

Mike looked shell shocked when he got off the phone. "Do you think we should go in?"

"No, I don't think we should. The doctor said it's just a precaution. Your dad needs to rest and he'd try to stay awake if we were there. Let him sleep tonight and we'll go in tomorrow morning."

We called Mike's brother and told him of the latest development, and then called Rodger's brother with the news as well. Both were concerned but were reassured when told he was moved to ICU as a precaution.

Two hours later the doctor called again. "Does your father have a living will?" he asked Mike.

"Yes. What's wrong?"

"Do you have the power to make medical decisions for your father?"

"Yes. I have medical power of attorney. What's going on?"

"As a precaution, I need to ask. If your father's condition worsens, do you want us to put him on a respirator?"

"I need more information before I answer that," Mike insisted. "What happens when you put someone on a respirator and why would you do it?"

"A person is put on a respirator when he or she can't breathe on their own. Sometimes it's done for a short time to allow the patient to breathe while his lungs heal from illness or trauma, or after some types of surgery. The problem with the respirator isn't hooking a patient up to it. It's making the decision to disconnect if the patient is incapable of surviving without it."

"When someone is brain dead, you mean."

"Yes."

"And you think that could happen to my father?"

"He's not in danger now but he's very ill. If he stops breathing, we aren't going to have time to call you to find out what your wishes are. I'm asking now so you can have some input. What does your father want?"

"I need to think about this," Mike answered. "I want to talk to my brother and my wife. I'll call you back."

"What do you think I should do?" he asked me.

"I think this is a decision you and your brother need to make."

"We will, but talking to you will help me think it through."

"I think that he's had a long life, much of it far more difficult than any of us will ever realize, and he deserves to die free of pain. If he were my father, I'd want him to be spared any unnecessary intervention."

"You'd say no to the respirator."

"I'd say no. We had to deal with this question when Mom was unresponsive for four days. All five of us agreed that she wouldn't want to be put on a machine. It was hard to say the words, but I believe it helped her more than a machine could have. "

He sighed. "This is too hard."

"I know." I took his hand in mine. I wish …"

"I know," he answered, reaching for the phone. "I know."

And he did know. Do not resuscitate, or DNR, are not words you ever want to say, but there are moments when it's the most loving thing a person can do.

After speaking with his brother and his uncle, Mike called the doctor and told him not to use a respirator just to maintain a semblance of life.

When we went in to see him the next day, he wasn't even aware we were there. He looked far weaker than he had been when he was admitted.

How much more can he take?

As we were turning to leave, he shifted slightly in his sleep and his eyes opened just for a moment. He looked directly at us.

He's still there, I thought. *He's not ready to go yet.*

"'Everyone has a destiny,' he told me one day shortly after my mother died," Mike said. "'When it's your time you go, no need to worry about it.'"

It wasn't his time and he really didn't have to worry. Mike and I had done it for him. The issue of the respirator never came up again, and he began to slowly improve.

The memory of that months-long ordeal stayed with me, and because of it, no matter what he said, I'd never let him take responsibility for his medicine again.

I stopped at his room on my way downstairs and listened at the door. Relieved to hear him snoring, I went on about my day. I started a load of laundry and tidied up the house, dusting and making the beds while thinking about what to make for dinner, eventually deciding to thaw a couple of steaks to cook on the grill. Mike and I would have them on the deck with a crisp salad and baked potatoes. Then I scanned the refrigerator to see what was available for Rodger's lunch. Seeing that his supplies were running low, I took out a package of chicken legs and put them in a roasting pan with some chopped onion and popped them into the oven. I peeled a couple of potatoes and put them on to boil, mixed up a batch of instant pudding, put it in individual serving bowls, and placed them in the refrigerator to set. Then I took out a bag of frozen broccoli and put the icy vegetables in the steamer and set the timer for ten minutes. While all that was cooking, I diced some apples, mixed in some sugar and cinnamon and put them into a pie pan. After topping them with ground cookie crumbs and a little butter,

I added that pan to the oven with the chicken. By the time Rodger came down again, everything would be cooked, cooled, and placed in resealable containers on his side of the refrigerator.

Sadly, he could no longer be trusted to use the stove. His short-term memory was getting bad. Twice he'd left food cooking on the stove, gone up to his room, and gone to sleep. We were lucky that one of us discovered what he'd done in time, and that the only damage done was to a couple of pots.

"I can't let you use the stove anymore," I told him after the second incident. "I'm afraid you'll forget again. You could burn the house down."

"I'll try not to," he answered sadly. "I can cook."

"No, not anymore. I'm home all the time now and I like to cook. It's safer this way."

"I can use the microwave," he insisted. "I can eat leftovers."

I agreed he could heat things up using the microwave, and every couple of days I cooked the foods I knew he liked and put them in the refrigerator, making sure that when he went looking for his leftovers, there was always a fresh supply of healthy food waiting for him.

I'd just folded the last item of laundry when I heard the telltale squeak of the floorboard outside his bathroom. It was lunchtime by then. I should have expected to hear him moving around, but I was deep in thought when he came out of his room. The noise surprised me and took me back again to the hospital and how close we had come to losing him.

Chapter 8

Mike knew immediately that something was wrong when I arrived home from the hospital the night I discovered Rodger was off his medication again.

"What's happened?" he asked before I had a chance to speak.

There was no hint of his usual warm smile when he greeted me. Once the words were spoken, he pressed his lips together so tightly they nearly disappeared, and the faint lines across his forehead grew into deep furrows.

"You better hope your face doesn't freeze like that," I tried to joke. "I need a hug."

"Me too," he admitted, opening his arms wide, inviting me to enter the safest place I know on earth. We stood like that for several minutes, enjoying the comforting warmth of the embrace, drawing strength from one another.

"What's wrong?" he asked, softer this time. "Are you all right?"

"I am, but your dad's not. I'll tell you all about it in a minute, but first I need a sniff."

I put my head on his shoulder and inhaled deeply. He smiled then. There's something about his scent that calms me, and I get as close to him as I can when worried or upset. He doesn't understand it, but he knows it works and has stopped questioning it. Sometimes I do it just for pure pleasure—and he's okay with that too.

"Do you want a cup of tea?" he asked, stepping out of the embrace.

"Yes, please, and something to eat if there's anything that won't take too much effort."

"I've got it covered, Babe."

He touched a few buttons on the microwave and heated the cup of water that was already waiting for me, tea bag in place. Then he went to the oven and removed a plate of warm chicken, mashed potatoes, and corn.

"You are my hero," I said, tears suddenly welling up in my eyes.

"Then why are you crying?"

After taking several sips of tea and a couple of bites of dinner, I went over all that had happened with Rodger and told him about the meeting I insisted on.

"I can't believe this. They tell us how wonderful their computerized record system is, allowing everyone involved with a patient to view his full record, and then they don't read it. What's the use?"

Before I had a chance to respond, the phone rang.

True to her word, the night nurse had contacted the patient advocate and told her how she stepped in and allowed Rodger to feed himself, causing him to choke and throw up. She also told her about my concerns that he'd not been taking his Zyprexa.

"Mrs. Carducci, I do apologize for the misunderstandings that concern you, but please be aware that everyone involved with your father-in-law's care wants what's best for him."

"My husband and I appreciate that. We also know that his case is complicated. He has a lot of doctors and he takes a lot of medication. That's why it's critical that everyone talk to each other and understand what his unique needs are."

"I agree," she said. "I've spoken with his medical doctor, his psychiatrist, and the charge nurse responsible for him on the ward. Can you meet with them and with me tomorrow morning at 10:30?"

"We'll be there."

After giving me directions to the conference room, she apologized again for the miscommunication and said goodbye.

"I take it that was the hospital," Mike said when I hung up the phone.

"Yes, the meeting is scheduled for tomorrow morning. I'm sorry I didn't think to ask if you could be there before agreeing to the time. I'm so tired I'm not thinking straight."

"Don't worry. I'm going with you." He picked up the phone, called his boss, and arranged to have the day off.

The only unfamiliar face in the room was that of the patient advocate. After introducing herself to us, she went over the events of the previous day and explained, for the record, why we were all there. In addition, seated around the table were Rodger's psychiatrist, his doctor of record for the duration of his current admission, and a nursing supervisor. The doctor spoke first, giving everyone an overview of his treatment since Rodger's admission with pneumonia, including a report on the results of an imaging test that had been done using a camera to film what happened when he tried to swallow. The test clearly showed that when he ate or drank, the food or liquid would collect at the base of his throat, causing him to choke and cough. He'd have to take small bites and chew thoroughly or risk aspirating, which would result in recurring bouts of pneumonia.

A theory was beginning to form in my mind, but I decided to wait a bit before mentioning it. I wanted to hear what the others had to say.

The next one to speak up was his psychiatrist. Mike and I were well acquainted with him, since we saw him regularly with Rodger.

"I was told you think he's not taking his Zyprexa." He directed his comment toward me.

"I'm convinced of it."

"What makes you say that?"

"The first thing I noticed was the involuntary movements of his head and arms. Then he told the nurses I was poisoning him. He said they were all in on it. He said we had to do what the boss told us to do, and when I asked him who the boss was, he said 'the government.' He said they know all about you even before you're born, and they know where to find you."

"He actually said that? He told you he believes the government is making you poison him?"

"Not only did he say that, but one of the nurses said something that made things worse. When she heard him say the government is the boss and we had to do what they say, she told him he was right. A sane person would know she meant that she works in a VA hospital and so her boss is the government, but he didn't understand it that way." I shook my head in disbelief at the implied ignorance of his case in what she'd said.

"Doctor, you and I have seen one another so often over the last several months that you're probably sick of looking at me. I tried to tell you over and over again that something was wrong. I described the same symptoms to you and everyone else we came into contact with and no one recognized what was happening until he had a full-blown psychotic break. He was so far gone by the time we got him in here we were told that he'd probably never be released. Arrangements were being made for long-term care. Then, out of the blue, we received a call telling us he'd been released and to come and pick him up by the end of the day.

"For eight weeks we were told one thing, and then all of a sudden someone we never spoke with before tells us he's well enough to come home. When we questioned the sudden change in diagnosis, it was suggested that we were protesting because we didn't want him back. That wasn't true then and it isn't true now. We asked what had brought about the sudden change in plans, and I believe that only one person told us the truth. Mike spoke with someone on the sixth floor and was told that they tried to place him in long-term care but the facility was full. He told him that this hospital is not a long-term care facility for the mentally ill, and Rodger had to be discharged. I believe it was at that point that someone decided to sedate him and send him home. If he ended up back in here, so be it."

When the advocate started to dispute that, I cut her off.

"I know no one in this hospital will admit to what I'm suggesting. I don't think anyone in this room would condone it, but I believe it's true. What's worse is that he was sick when they released him. He coughed all the way home and all through the night. He couldn't eat or drink anything. Every time he tried, he'd cough so violently he'd turn blue, and he was so listless he could barely function. When he continued to get worse, we had no choice but to bring him back.

Then the nurse in the emergency room lectured me for doing it. She said she knew we'd rather have him in the hospital than at home, but the hospital was not a good place for him. It was full of germs and he could get worse. At that point I was so angry I demanded she explain how I could take care of him at home. He couldn't eat, he couldn't drink anything, his blood oxygen level was dangerously low, and he was barely conscious.

"'Never mind,' she said, 'just forget it.'

"Forget it? Believe me there is no way I'm about to forget that! He ended up back in the emergency room because he didn't get the right care while he was here. And he didn't get the right care, not because the people on the sixth floor are callous and unfeeling, he didn't get proper care because no one saw the whole picture. Now the same thing is happening in reverse. Upstairs, the mental health professionals weren't monitoring his physical well-being. Now that he's off that floor, no one here is watching his mental state."

"I don't think I'd go that far," the nurse said.

"Look, I'm not here to point fingers or accuse anyone of ill-intent. I know all of you are very busy and you have hundreds of patients for whom you are responsible. I have it easier, I only have one. He's my family and my full-time job, and as part of that job it's up to me to make sure he gets the care he needs. In order for that to happen, you people have to communicate with one another and with me on a regular basis. I'd hate for you to think of us as the 'screaming Carduccis,' but if that's what it takes to get you to listen, then that's what we'll do."

His advocate smiled at the "screaming Carduccis" remark and assured me it wouldn't be necessary.

"Your father-in-law is lucky to have the two of you in his corner," she said, acknowledging both Mike and me. "As hard as we try, sometimes things get overlooked. We're only human, and it's important for families to be involved. You're the ones who see them every day and are in the best position to recognize changes."

"Well, the other part of that," Mike said, "is that you people have to listen to what we tell you. My father was clearly not doing well long before he was admitted."

"We can't change what happened before this meeting," the advocate answered. "But you did the right thing coming here today, and now that we know what the problem is we can take steps to fix it."

"That's what we came for," Mike told her, rising and reaching out to shake hands with each person at the table, "and I'm pleased to hear we're all in agreement."

"Thank you," she said. "Feel free to call me if you need anything in the future."

"Oh you can be sure of that," he answered, a rarely seen but very effective steely glint punctuating his remark. "But, knowing my wife, I hope it isn't necessary."

Remembering my thoughts from the doctor's report at the beginning of the meeting, I had one more question. "Doctor, tests were being run to find out if Rodger's had a small stroke. If he had, that could explain his swallowing problems. Are the results back yet?"

"Yes, and there is no indication he had a stroke."

"Is it possible it's a symptom of Parkinson's disease?"

"Difficulty swallowing can be a symptom of Parkinson's, but it says in your father-in-law's chart the he was seen by a neurologist shortly before he was admitted and there was no indication of the disease. Why are you asking me this now?"

"I know what the neurologist said, but there are other signs, like the hand tremor, slow, sometimes slurred speech, the awkward way he moves sometimes. It runs in his family. I want to make sure we aren't missing something."

"The neurologist you saw is very good, and the symptoms you describe can all be attributed to his long history of taking antipsychotic drugs. I'd listen to the specialist and not add another problem to what we're already dealing with. Let's get him over the pneumonia and home where he belongs."

I thanked him and everyone else for their time and the meeting ended.

On the way home, I apologized to Mike for taking over and hardly giving him a chance to speak.

"I didn't mind," he assured me. "You were doing fine on your own, and you spend more time with my dad than I do. Plus, they need to know that you're the one they have to deal with. You did great, my love, no need to apologize at all."

Three weeks later, Rodger had improved enough to go home. The crisis was over, and I was eager to get on with everyday life. What I didn't understand was how demanding everyday life was about to become.

Chapter 9

Whoever wrote in Rodger's chart, "Intelligence is estimated to be below average," was very wrong. Rodger was a serious scholar, described by his younger brother as, "a bookish teenager who took advanced degrees in mathematics and literature at an early age. He tried to help me with my schoolwork, but what came easy for him was very hard for me. He'd try to help me with algebra but he'd go so fast I couldn't keep up."

Rodger graduated Summa Cum Laude from college. He spoke six languages, including Latin, Italian, French, German, English, and some Yugoslavian. Remarkable for a man who grew up on a farm in Tornimparte, Italy.

"We raised or grew everything we needed to live. We grew our own wheat, and at harvest time all the farmers would go in together and rent a threshing machine. It would take a long time before all the work was finished, but we did it. Then the women make pasta and bread. Every day, my mother, she get up, make the polenta, and go to church. Then she come home and work all day. She cook, she clean, she open a store in our house. She do all she can to make money. My father, he's in America working in the coal mines. Life is hard for everybody."

The family farm included a vineyard, and their homemade wine was sold in the store alongside the produce and bread to keep the farm running and the family clothed and fed.

While Rodger kept the books for both the vineyard and the store, his younger brother helped more in the fields, with the harvesting, and in the gardens. Rodger also did his share of hard work. His shoulder was scarred from a deep cut he received while carrying heavy loads of grapes down a steep hill to be crushed and fermented into wine.

"It hurt like hell, but there was nothing I could do. I had come too far. I couldn't go back, I had to keep going."

The cut to his shoulder must have been very deep. It damaged a vein in his wrist that remained enlarged and sensitive the rest of his life.

The more I learned about him, the more I admired him. There I was, caring for an extraordinary man whose native intelligence was far beyond my own. He had struggled to help his family survive while still little more than a boy, only to be struck down by an illness few people understand, the treatment of which left him with huge gaps in his memory, making it impossible for him to do anything but menial labor. It became obvious to me that bits of his superior intelligence remained. Even after all the years of being drugged and probed and experimented upon, he'd managed to build a life and raise a family. Now, in his old age, the deficits were mounting. Sadly, the blessings of his youth, combined with the severity of his losses, would leave him aware enough to know something was very wrong but unable to figure out what it was or why he couldn't do the one thing he wanted most—take care of himself. The lengths to which he'd go in order to prove he could do it would result in seven years of cat-and-mouse games that tried us both and bound us together through shared experiences that were at times funny, but far too often were frustrating and confusing for both of us.

"It don't make sense," was a phrase he used almost daily. More often than not, I had to agree.

Chapter 10

After Rodger had lunch and his afternoon walk, he was ready for a nap. I used the quiet time each day to shop for groceries and run any errands that needed to be done. That day I decided there was nothing on my to-do list that couldn't wait, but I needed to get out of the house. With no plan in mind, I opened the windows in the car, allowing the cool breeze to ruffle my hair as I took in several deep breaths. Letting the air out slowly in an attempt to ease the tension in my back and shoulders, I knew where I needed to go.

There were only two cars in the church parking lot when I pulled in, but considering it was a weekday afternoon, that wasn't surprising. After dipping my fingers into the holy water font and making the sign of the cross, I slipped into a pew near the front of the church. For several moments I simply sat there, taking in the lingering aroma of incense, candle wax, and furniture polish. That familiar smell never fails to invoke memories of weddings, baptisms, first communion celebrations, and Sister Mary Josephine, my fourth-grade teacher, who, with her back as straight and her steps as measured as any four-star general, led her class to Mass every day before lunch.

"Our Father, who art in Heaven,… " I prayed, the words taking on a new importance as tears of frustration and guilt streamed down my face. "Thy kingdom come. Thy will be done …"

All right, God, if it is Your will that I take care of my father-in-law, I'm happy to do it. But You have to help me. I'm new at this, and I'm afraid I'm not doing it very well. He's a sick old man, and he's not trying to be difficult. I know that. So why do I feel so angry?

"… And forgive us our trespasses, as we forgive those who trespass against us…. but deliver us from evil … " I sobbed, my heart breaking for both of us. Why couldn't I be stronger?

"Help me to be more patient and understanding. Guide me to make the right decisions when it comes to his care. Help me find the right words to soothe him when he's confused and frightened. Please take the anger away. It frightens me. It weakens me, and I need to be strong to do this. I don't want to let Mike down, and I can't let Rodger down. He has nowhere else to go. Please, hold me in your love and light and show me the path you want me to take. Amen."

My prayer complete, I struggled to stop crying, but the harder I tried the harder the tears flowed. Just as I began to fear they'd never end, exhaustion and embarrassment forced me to gain control of myself. *Get a grip*, I scolded myself. *You've had a good cry, and it's time to go home.*

I'd left my purse in the car and had nothing to mop up the watery mess I'd made of myself, leaving me with no choice other than to wipe my nose on my sleeve. I didn't notice the near-silent approach of the only other person in the church until a tiny elderly woman, dressed all in black, touched my shoulder and handed me a bunch of tissues.

"God bless you," she whispered as she turned and walked away.

Yes, God bless me. I sure do need it.

Chapter 11

The whine of the sanding tool the podiatrist was using to file down Rodger's thick, infected toenails set up a sympathetic hum in the fillings in my back teeth. My mouth went dry, and I could feel my toes curling inside my shoes. I had been shocked to discover the condition of his feet when I happened to enter his room shortly after he'd taken a shower one day. He was sitting on the side of the bed, struggling to keep his balance while putting on his socks.

"Do you want some help?"

"No, I can do it," he replied, trying to get the opening of a sock over his foot, only to have it catch on a very long, curved toenail.

"Let me look at your feet," I said, moving closer.

I was appalled at what I found. Every nail was an ugly shade of yellow-brown. They were so curled and long I knew they must cause him pain when he walked.

"How long have your feet been like this?"

"What's the matter? They're just toenails. When you get old, they grow."

"Do they hurt?"

"Not too much. I try to cut them with the clippers but it won't work."

"They're infected. I'll make an appointment for you to see the doctor. Maybe he can give us some medicine to soften them so they can be trimmed."

"This is caused by a fungus," the podiatrist explained. "It's not unusual to see it in the elderly. I'll file them down and trim them for him and then I'll see him every three months to keep the fungal regrowth under control. And I'm going to order custom-made shoes for him. They'll have a deeper toe box so the thick nails don't cramp his toes."

"I've seen treatments advertised on TV for toenail fungus. Can't we use that? If not, I understand there's an oral medication that can be used to treat it."

"I don't advise using either. The topical treatments can burn the sensitive skin around the nail, and the pills can have an adverse effect on his liver. It's better to bring him in and let me trim them as needed. They were in very bad shape this time, and I had to trim them back a lot. There are some raw areas around three of his toes that will have to be treated for the next few days. I'm ordering some supplies for you take home, and I want you to bring him back in a week so I can check them."

Soon Rodger and I were on our way again. He, muttering that he didn't need new shoes, it was a waste of money, and me, carrying a box with all the stuff the pharmacist handed me when we stopped to pick up the supplies the doctor ordered. Sterile saline, antifungal cream, peroxide, sterile pads, and a box of cloth tubing of some sort. I was told to have him soak his foot in warm water and sterile saline for twenty minutes, then apply the peroxide, followed by the antifungal cream, wrap the toes in the sterile pads, and use the cloth tube to hold the bandage in place. Treatments were to be done three times a day for four days. If I saw any sign of infection in his toes or foot, I was to call for an appointment right away. Otherwise, the doctor would see him in a week.

Already his days were tightly scheduled around his meals and medications, but I fitted in these latest treatments around them. The first day wasn't a problem. I followed the doctor's orders precisely. One treatment after his morning walk, another while he watched his favorite afternoon programs, and the last after supper. On the second day one of his obsessions kicked in and I had to figure out a way to work around it. I called moments like these creative problem-solving on the run.

When he first came to live with us, the only things he asked us to buy for him were Milk of Magnesia and prune juice. He had prescriptions for stool softeners and laxatives issued by his former doctors and continued by his new doctor. He constantly complained of constipation, greeting everyone he spoke to, including strangers, with "Hello. How's everything? My bowels don't move." If he did happen to go, he made sure he told them about that as well, in great detail. It soon became clear he was taking far too much of the stuff. Every day, in the morning and at midday, he'd drink a large glass of prune juice, followed by Milk of Magnesia. Often he'd wait a few moments after taking it, look at his watch, and take some more. A few moments later he'd do it again. One day, after just telling me he'd had a bowel movement, I saw him drink another large glass of prune juice and reach for the Milk of Magnesia.

"Why are you taking that? " I asked.

"For the constipation," he said.

"But you just went."

"That don't count. It was all liquid."

That's when I knew I had to do something. No matter how we tried to explain it to him, he wouldn't accept that it was the laxatives that were causing his problem. The more he took, the worse it got—and the more he worried—resulting in a vicious cycle that was interfering in his normal bodily functions. His psychiatrist said that it's not unusual for a schizophrenic to keep track of what goes in and out of his body. In his mind, solid food was going in but nothing solid was coming out. That meant something was very wrong. Once I began to limit his access to prune juice and Milk of Magnesia, and started monitoring his use of laxatives, he started showing signs of stress. He paced and muttered to himself and began making frequent trips to the bathroom where he'd sit for hours, waiting for something to happen. I hated to see him like that, but I had to ease him off the stuff. His doctor tried to help by telling him that taking too many laxatives could interfere with his other medications and land him back in the hospital. He wasn't buying it. When I wouldn't give in, he complained to Mike, and when Mike backed me up, he called him one of the worst insults he could think of.

"You're nothing but a dictator! You're another Mussolini, that's what you are!"

Later, after Rodger calmed down and we were getting ready for bed, Mike looked over at me and shook his head. "Mussolini? Now I'm Mussolini?"

I couldn't hold it in any longer. The giggles I'd been trying hard to stifle came rolling out. "The Mussolini of laxatives!" I laughed harder. "You Fascist poop dictator!"

Mike looked at me in confusion for a moment, and then the hilarity of the situation hit him and he was laughing as hard as I was. I laughed so hard I got the hiccups, and that made us laugh even more. We ended up rolling on the bed, laughter feeding more laughter, until we were exhausted.

"Oh wow, I needed that," I said when I was finally able to catch my breath.

"Me too," Mike agreed. "I don't know how you do it every day. He's so damned stubborn. I'm glad I'm not like that."

"Right." I poked him the ribs. "Me either. I'm not stubborn. I'm determined."

"Yes, dear," Mike said with a grin. "Do you think you can determine to keep loving me through all this?"

"Sure, if you can determine to come over here and give me a kiss."

"Sure thing, Babe." He enveloped me in his arms and kissed me. "I know you're struggling a lot more than you're letting on. I leave you here to bear the brunt of the work while I go to the office. I'm almost ashamed to admit I'm relieved I can get away for a while each day. I don't have your patience or ability to come up with new ways to deal with his quirks. But I feel so damn guilty all the time. Tell me what to do to make it better for you."

"Spend some time with him when you are home. Give me a chance to get out of the house for a while and not have to watch the clock all the time. And laugh with me more often. I really need that."

"I will," he promised. "And someday I'll find a way to show you how much I appreciate what you do."

Over the next few weeks I gradually weaned Rodger off most of the laxatives, and his body began to work on its own. He was not happy. He still insisted he needed laxatives and resented me for taking them from him.

"You don't understand. I eat. I have to have laxatives."

"Your body is working fine. You told me you went this morning."

"No I didn't," he insisted. "It's been a week, two weeks, a month. I'm going to explode."

"You went this morning," I insisted right back.

How in hell was I going to convince him that he really did go, and what was my life was coming to when my daily interactions with another person consisted of arguments over shit?

"I don't forget nothing. You don't understand."

"You're right. I don't understand," I said. "Why do you keep creating a problem where there isn't one? Don't we have enough to deal with already? You eat. You go to the bathroom like everybody else. I think you like making things difficult. It makes you feel important. 'Look what I can make her do,' you say to yourself. No wonder Shirley was angry all the time. You drove her crazy." I walked away, afraid of what I might say next.

"Shirley always had to have things her way. You couldn't tell her nothing," he said.

"I'm glad you aren't like that," I answered with a wry laugh, the tension going out of me as I realized how silly the exchange had been.

I tried to keep in mind that his reality was different than mine—and it was his I had deal with. I had to find a way to convince him he went to the bathroom regularly.

The next day I gave him a small notebook with his name on it. I divided the pages into columns labeled BM, Date, and Name. I explained that we were going to use it to keep track of his bowel movements. Every time he went, he was to put a check mark in the column labeled BM then sign his name and date it. It would help us keep track of what was happening or not happening, and make sure he didn't explode. He liked the idea and never missed an entry in his log. Soon he began expanding his reports with comments like, big splash, all out, or two small pieces. If he went more than two days without an entry, I'd slip a laxative into the applesauce he took with his medication. It helped a lot but it didn't make the problem go away entirely. He began spending a lot of time in the bathroom, anticipating his next bowel movement.

I knew I was in for trouble when I realized he'd been in and out of the bathroom all morning, much of the time with door open. Earlier, when I'd walked past on the way to get dressed, I'd seen him sitting on the toilet looking out the window. On my way back, I saw him stand and look into the bowl, shake his head, and sit down again. Seeing me look in, he reached over and firmly closed the door.

And keep it closed, I thought. I didn't need to see that again anytime soon.

Later, when it was time to treat his toes, he was still in there.

"Rodger, come out of the bathroom. I have to take care of your foot."

"No! I can't. It's the constipation again. I have to wait until I go."

"Can't you come out long enough to get your foot taken care of?"

"No!"

Rather than argue and get us both in a tizzy, I decided to work around the problem. I gathered up the basin I used to soak his foot and all the other supplies I needed and knocked on the door.

"Put a towel over your lap. I'm coming in."

"I can't reach it," he said.

I opened the door partway, reached around it, and handed him the towel I planned to use to dry his foot before applying the medication. Then I got another one from the linen closet and asked if he was ready.

"Ready," he answered, opening the door to let me in.

I placed his foot in the warm water bath and told him I'd be back in twenty minutes. When the time was up, I went in to complete the treatment. I was on my knees in front of him, applying the antifungal cream, when I heard a faint plopping noise.

"Something just came out," he said. "There goes another piece," he said a moment later.

I kept my head down, trying to work faster and keep a straight face so I could get out of there as soon as possible. I finally got the gauze pad on and the mesh wrapper securely in place after several tries.

He grunted and bore down. "Ahh, big splash out. All done," he said, reaching for the toilet paper roll.

"Wait a minute," I said, trying to stifle a laugh. "Let me give you some privacy before you do that."

As I gathered up my supplies and the basin and made a hasty retreat, I wondered if the entire exercise had been a joke God was playing on me. If I had waited a few more minutes, would he have achieved splashdown in time to avoid the whole towel-over-his-lap scene? Or was this some weird penance I had to pay for the times I messed up in my life?

And people had asked me what I was going to do all day when I quit my job. Wouldn't they be surprised if I told them?

"Baby!" I answered when the phone rang. I knew from the caller ID that it was Mike letting me know he was on his way home.

"I love you," he said.

"That's the best thing I've heard all day."

"Well, you might hear it again. What a bad day I've had. Meeting after meeting and I got nothing done." Mike sighed.

"Oh no you don't. I know your day was much better than mine," I interrupted. "Your father was having one of his sit-down strikes in the bathroom today."

"Sit-down strikes?"

"You know, where he sits on the toilet waiting for the big event."

"Oh boy."

"That's not the best part. Remember, I have to take care of his foot three times a day. He refused to come out, so I was on my knees in the bathroom treating his toe fungus while he gave me a running report about what was coming out of his butt."

"Oh my God! You win." Mike laughed. "Nothing that happened to me can come close to topping that. You, my dear, are a saint," he said, still laughing.

"I don't know about that, but I can use a drink. Come home and have a glass of wine with me."

"Sounds like a plan. I'm on my way."

Chapter 12

"Since none of the kids will be here this year, I'd like to do something special for the three of us," I said a few weeks before Easter.

"What do you have in mind?" Mike asked.

"I think it would be nice to make a special dinner for Rodger and serve it in the dining room. We can use the good china and silverware. He'll be the guest of honor and sit at the head of the table. I'll roast a chicken and make a sauce for gnocchi. I know that's one of his favorite foods. I'll serve it with a side salad and some wine for us and sparkling grape juice for him. For dessert I'll make an apple pie."

"I think that's a great idea," Mike said, licking his lips in anticipation. "I love your sauce."

I looked forward to the holiday with growing enthusiasm. I hoped Rodger would enjoy a change in routine that didn't involve seeing a doctor. I bought him a small Easter basket and filled it with sugar-free candies and a small chocolate bunny, also sugar free. He didn't have diabetes and his blood sugar readings were always well within normal range, but he had been overweight in the past and one of his doctors had mentioned he should cut back on sugar. From then on he requested sugar-free treats. I wondered why that suggestion stuck with him, while repeated instruction about other things, like the need to take his medication every day, were not only ignored but openly defied.

On Easter morning the aroma of pasta sauce and roasting chicken wafted through the house. A beautiful apple pie rested on the kitchen counter. I hummed "Here Comes Peter Cotton Tail" as I adjusted my best tablecloth before going to the china cabinet and getting three place settings, consisting of dinner plate, salad plate, and bread plate. After carefully placing the proper utensils next to the plates, I added a water glass and a delicate wine goblet and stepped back to admire the table. Mike had folded cloth napkins into delicate winged swans to be placed in the center of the dinner plates. Silver candlesticks flanked a beautiful flower arrangement that complimented the décor perfectly. Just before calling the men to dinner, I'd cut the pie and place three pieces on matching dessert plates, ready to be served when the time came.

Rodger had looked pleased when Mike and I went into his sitting room and presented him with his Easter basket that morning.

"Happy Easter," we greeted him.

"Happy Easter, he replied. "What's all this?"

"It's some Easter candy to sweeten your day," I said.

"They don't have Easter candy in the old country. Easter is a religious day. Everybody goes to church," Rodger said.

"It's a religious holiday for people here too," I explained. "But we also have the traditional Easter baskets."

"Do I have to go to church?" he asked. "I only go to church when somebody marries or dies."

"You don't have to go to church if you don't want to," Mike assured him. "Enjoy your candy and join us later for dinner in the dining room. Bobbi is making a special dinner."

"Who's coming? Do I have to take a shower?"

"No one is coming. It will be the three of us. But it would be nice if you took a shower. You'll be nice and clean for dinner."

"I don't need to take a shower to eat. I don't need special food. I eat anything"

"We know you'll eat anything," I said. "But on holidays we like to have a special meal. And you don't have to take a shower today but you will have to take one soon. You need it. I'll call you when dinner's ready."

I could tell he was curious about what was going on when he came down to go for a walk and saw the table set in the dining room. He didn't say anything but spent several minutes looking at it on his way out.

Even the weather was cooperating. The air was warm and the

sun was shining. After his walk, Rodger sat on his bench in the front yard and watched the birds flitting between the two feeders hanging from the tree he watched grow from the day we moved in.

He had become a fixture in the neighborhood, taking his three daily walks. He knew when people were moving in and when a house was listed for sale. He kept track of who had dogs and if they barked when he passed by or not. He always let me know when anyone planted something new in their yard and when the Christmas decorations went up. He rarely spoke to anyone, but he knew who lived where and could tell if they changed their routine in any way.

Despite his earlier protest, when I called the men to dinner, Rodger arrived freshly showered and shaved, wearing clean clothes and a shy smile.

"Sit here, Dad," Mike said as he pulled out the chair at the head of the table.

"Me, here?" he asked.

"Yes, you're the guest of honor today."

"Guest of honor. I'm not a guest of honor. I'm not special."

"You are to us," Mike and I said at the same time.

Rodger didn't speak as he filled his dish with chicken and pasta. Nor did he say anything when I passed him a plate of salad and offered him some toasted garlic bread from the napkin-covered serving dish.

"Before we eat, let's have a toast. Your wine glass has sparkling grape juice so you can drink too," Mike told his father. "Happy Easter," he said, raising his glass. "And to Rodger," he added.

I lifted my glass to my father-in-law and repeated Mike's toast. "To Rodger. We're so pleased you joined us to celebrate today. You look very nice."

"Thank you," he said. Then he lifted his fork and began to eat. Everyone was quiet for several minutes, each lost in thought and enjoying the meal. When Rodger broke the silence and began to speak, Mike and I were stunned to see tears in his eyes.

"I never thought I'd have a meal like this, in a place like this. Everything is beautiful. The food, the dishes, flowers and candles, everything. I feel like a big shot."

Dabbing at this eyes with his napkin, he looked around the room pointing to the delicately carved chairs and the gleaming china cabinets. He took a few moments to gaze at the framed print hanging on the wall. "Dinner at the Ritz," it's called. In it is depicted a group of Victorian ladies dining in their finery at flower-laden tables on a summer afternoon.

"Beautiful ladies," he said. "Everything is nice. I never thought I'd have anything like this. I can't believe I'm going to die here. I was born in a big house, and I'm going to die in a big house. Thank you."

We didn't know what to say. We had never seen him so touched by anything. We didn't know he could be moved like that. We were grateful and humbled at the same time. Whatever happened in the future, no matter how hard things got, we'd always have this moment with him.

Chapter 13

"She's a drunk! She drinks, you know."

Mike stood in the entryway to the kitchen. He'd just come home from work. All day I'd hoped we could share a quiet evening for a change. For months, every time he walked in the door, I greeted him first with a hug and then a sigh of relief. I was so grateful he was home. I couldn't wait for him to catch his breath after the long commute before launching into a litany of things his father had said or done during the day. Too often I'd cry on his shoulder, worn out from trying to anticipate the old man's every need before it became an obsession. When I couldn't keep him calm or avoid another crisis or, God forbid, I got angry with him, I'd be overcome with guilt for failing both men. I couldn't accept it when Mike told me he was impressed with what I was able to accomplish with his father and that he found it hard to understand why I felt I was failing anyone.

Usually when he came home, his father was up in his sitting room watching TV. On a good day he'd step out long enough to say 'Hi. How's everything?" barely waiting for an answer before turning his back and returning to his couch to listen to the news. The fact that he was now sitting at the kitchen table, clearly agitated, meant something must have gone very wrong.

"What's going on?" Mike asked me.

"He's been waiting for you for over an hour."

I lifted an almost-empty glass of wine off the table and took a generous drink, my eyes never leaving my father-in-law's face.

"You see!" he pointed. "She drinks. She's a drunk. You think you know everything but you don't."

"What got him started?" Mike asked.

"I don't know. He woke up in a pretty good mood. He sat and talked with me for about two hours after his walk this morning. I thought we were going to have a good day and we did—right up until lunch.

"What happened then?"

"I reminded him he has three doctor's appointments tomorrow."

"Three?"

"His primary care doctor, the cardiologist, and a new one. They want him to see a specialist for an evaluation to determine if he has age-related dementia."

"And what good will it do? Will it change anything? We know he's affected and it's not going to get better."

"I don't know. I'll ask when I get there." I sighed again and took another sip of wine.

"He's upset about going to the doctor?"

"He's upset because when he lived in Pittsburgh he didn't have to go to the doctor so often. He's upset that he has to take a shower. He wants to take care of his medicine himself. He's a man and I'm only a woman. Women in the old country are second-class citizens and know their place. Shirley never went in to see the doctor with him. She stayed in the car and waited for him. He wants laxatives and Milk of Magnesia. He insists he's constipated when he's not, although I do agree that he's full of shit. Especially today. I listened to this all day long. First one thing then another, over and over, until finally he wore himself out. When I heard him snoring, I took a long, hot shower and decided to have a glass of wine and chill out for a bit. The next thing I knew, he was down here accusing me of being a drunk."

"She was probably a drunk when you married her. That's why she got divorced. I bet you didn't know that," Rodger said, shaking his head and pointing at the wine glass again. "I've been watching her. She had two glasses already. You leave me alone with an alcoholic all day. I can take care of myself."

"She drinks because you drive her crazy!" Mike snapped. "In fact, you're driving us both crazy right now, and I'm going to join her in having a glass of wine."

"See, she makes you drink too."

"No, if anyone makes me drink, it's you."

"So it's all my fault?"

"Yes. It's all your fault. We're trying our best to take care of you and all you do is bitch and complain. She cooks and cleans for you. She takes you to the doctor. She cares for you when you're sick. She puts up with your complaining day after day, and do you ever say thank you? No. You don't. You whine about laxatives and tell people you don't want to live here. What the hell is wrong with you? If you don't live here, where do you think you're going to go? Who will take care of you?"

"My brother will take care of me."

"Yeah, right. Your brother will take care of you. Where is he now? How many times has he been here to see you? You've been here five years. Sometimes he comes on your birthday and stops by a few days after Christmas, if you're lucky. He's not going to take you in. He's been to Italy to visit your family there more often than he's been here."

"He's a busy man, my brother."

"Yes, he's busy. I'm busy. Bobbi's busy. We're all busy. He's no busier than the rest of us. If he can go Italy for two weeks whenever he feels like it, he can drive for thirty minutes and come here. But he doesn't, does he? Why do you think that is, Dad? Could it be that it's easier to let us handle it than to offer any help? Could it be he knows you'll do the same thing there as you do here, and he's not willing to inconvenience himself to put up with it?"

"I'll call my other son. I can live with him."

"You think so? Stay right there. I'll get the phone for you. Hell, I'll even dial it for you. See what he says when you tell him you want to live with him. Where has he been all this time? Does he come to visit? Does he even call you on your birthday or Christmas? You want to leave here and live with him? You must be drunk, not her."

"I don't drink nothing. I take too much medicine. You're crazy, like her. You do anything she says. She's in charge of you and you don't know it."

"I don't mind. She's a smart woman. A good woman. At least I know enough to listen when someone who's smarter than me is looking out for me."

"Ah, it's no use talking to you. You don't listen. You're just like your mother. Can't tell you nothing. I'm going to my room. I'll tell the doctor, that's what I'll do. She drinks and you don't listen."

Relieved to see him go, Mike and I stared at one another for a few seconds, each shocked by the emotion that had come out in that exchange. Each of us was tired and frustrated and near the end of our rope. We all needed a break. The problem was, how could we make that happen?

"So would you like a glass of wine?" I asked.

"You open another bottle and I'll pour, once I get out of these work clothes and into something more comfortable. And who's delivering dinner tonight? I see you didn't cook anything. What were you doing all day? Oh, I forgot, you were sitting around drinking," Mike said with a twinkle in his eye, and added, "You should do it more often."

Rodger appeared to have settled down by the time I took him his last medication for the night. He made no mention of the earlier confrontation and even managed a tiny smile as he wished me goodnight.

I had a more difficult time putting the ugly scene behind me. How could things have gone so wrong when all we wanted was to create an environment where he'd be safe, comfortable, and happy? Later, as I listened to the loud snores emanating from my father-in-law's bedroom down the hall, I lay awake until almost dawn wondering how I could have responded better to him throughout the day. If I hadn't let his bad mood and negative comments get to me, I might not have had those two glasses of wine, setting him off again and making things worse for everyone.

Why can't I get it right? How many mistakes do I have to make before something I do, or fail to do, results in another crisis, one that he can't recover from? What will Mike think of me then? What if, in trying to save his father, I lose him?

Unfortunately, no matter how long I lay awake, neither prayer nor worry provided any answers. All I could do was resolve to carry on and do the best I could in the moment.

Brilliant, Bobbi! You do know the definition of insanity is doing the same thing over and over while expecting a different result, don't you? Which one is crazy now?

Finally, giving up on getting hit with a flash of insight, I pulled the covers up over my shoulders and snuggled up to Mike's back, in the hope his scent would sooth me to sleep before I had to get up and get ready for the trip to the VA hospital in the morning.

Chapter 14

"Who do we see today?" Rodger asked, as he we approached the hospital entrance. He'd asked the same question several times before we left the house and repeatedly during the forty-minute drive.

"First, your primary care doctor, Dr. Jameson, and then—"

"What time is the appointment?" he interrupted.

"Nine-thirty."

"Then I see who?" he asked.

Then you see your cardiologist, Dr. Keye, at 10:45."

"He says my heart will last twenty years. Every time he says the same thing. I don't want to live that long. I don't want to end up in a wheelchair. I'd rather be dead."

"Not so loud," I hushed him as a man in a wheelchair came around the corner.

I hoped he hadn't heard Rodger's comments. I'd seen him around the hospital every time we were there. He appeared to be one of the long-term residents. Sometimes he was fully dressed, and other times he'd be in pajamas and a robe tooling around the halls. I'd seen him in the commissary and the barber shop and sometimes in the lobby reading a book. Both his legs were missing below the knee. He often joked with the guards at the main desk, and always had a smile and a glance for any pretty women who passed by. I thought about pointing out that he seemed to be happy, despite the wheelchair, but I knew it would do no good. Rodger wouldn't believe me, and I didn't know how the man felt. Was his smile a fleeting ruse he used to try to convince himself he was living and not merely existing? Did he have family who loved him and visited often, or was he there because he had no choice, doomed to marking time in a warehouse of injured and forgotten men and women?

"After that, we're done," Rodger said.

"After that you go to see a new doctor. He's going to test your memory."

"Why? I remember everything. I don't need a test. I remember Shirley. You couldn't tell her anything. She had to be right. I remember lots of things. Tell them not to waste their money. I remember what I need to remember."

"Dr. Jameson ordered the test, so we have to go. It won't take long and it won't hurt. The doctor will ask you some questions and then we can go home."

"Too many questions. It's none of their business if I forget. I remember what I need to remember. I remember Shirley. What doctor are we going to see today?"

The visit with the primary doctor and the cardiologist were routine and revealed nothing new. His weight was down a little more but remained in normal range. His vital signs were holding, and he insisted to both doctors that he was fine and I worried too much. By the time those appointments were over it was almost time for lunch, and we had a two-hour wait before he'd be seen by the new doctor.

I led Rodger to the cafeteria, hoping he wouldn't notice it was twenty minutes earlier than he was used to eating. No such luck. As soon as we approached the entrance, he looked at his watch.

"It's not time to eat. I eat at 12:00. It's now 11:40." He stopped walking and stood in place, looking at the people already eating or carrying trays of food to the tables scattered throughout the room. "It's not time to eat." He swayed a bit as anxiety began to flow through him.

"It's okay, you don't have to eat yet," I said. "We can sit at one of the tables and wait until it's time."

He began to relax immediately. "That's right. We can wait. I eat at 12:00. It's 11:42. What doctor do I see today?"

At precisely 12:00, he rose from his chair and joined the cafeteria line. Once he had a tray and a set of plastic silverware, he inched his way past the array of food, filling his plate with mashed potatoes, green beans, corn, beets, and beef stew. He added vanilla pudding for dessert and filled a paper cup halfway with warm diet soda.

"Is that all you're going to eat?" he asked, eyeing my cup of chicken soup and plate of salad.

"That's all need," I replied.

I was happy he had selected soft foods that were less likely to send him into a coughing fit when he overfilled his mouth. These trips to the hospital were his only opportunity to choose what he would eat. I knew it wasn't good for him, but he enjoyed it and I didn't want to embarrass him. He often accused me of treating him like a child. To select his food for him in public would make it worse. I had no appetite for cafeteria food and wondered how so many people in the health industry could eat these overprocessed, oversalted, fat-saturated meals every day. No wonder so many of them were overweight.

Soon after he finished lunch and cleared away his tray, it was time to meet the new doctor. I wondered as we rode the elevator to the third floor what new issues would be revealed by the tests and what impact they'd have on him. I said a silent prayer that this time the news would be, if not good, at least not devastating.

How much more of himself can he lose? I asked God

"Who do we see today?" Rodger asked as the elevator door slid open.

Before I had a chance to answer, we were greeted by a smiling young man in a white lab coat. "Come in, Mr. Carducci. How are you today? I'm Dr. Gregory and I'll be seeing you every three months from now on. And you must be his daughter-in-law, the lady who takes such good care of him," he said, turning to me.

"She worries too much," Rodger responded before I had a chance to say anything. "I don't need any more doctors. In Pittsburgh, I didn't have so many doctors."

"Don't worry Mr. Carducci. I'm not going to give you any shots or cause you pain. All I'm going to do is ask you some questions and have you do a few simple tasks, so I can see how your memory is working."

"I remember what I need to remember. I don't need tests. Who told you to see me? Did she call you?"

"Your primary care doctor made the appointment. Sometimes when people are older, they begin to have trouble remembering where they put things, what things are called, sometimes they even forget where they live and who their family members are."

"I know where I live. I know her. She's okay. She cooks. She cleans. My son married her. Sometimes she drinks wine."

"That's very good, Mr. Carducci. It shows me that you remember a lot of things. But, in case things change in the future, will you answer some questions for me today?"

"I have no choice. Ask your questions so I can go home. She worries too much."

"Where do you live?"

"Round Wall, Virginia."

The doctor looked to me for confirmation. "Round Hill," I said.

"Close enough." The doctor nodded approvingly. "Do you know your street address?"

"524110 Lavender Drive."

I nodded to indicate he was correct.

"Do you know where you are now?" the doctor continued.

"In the hospital answering your questions."

The doctor stifled a laugh at that response. "Let's move on. You're doing very well. I'm going to say three words and I want you to repeat them for me if you can. Are you ready?"

"Ready."

"Apple, book, hammer."

"Apple, book, … um, apple, book, … book, apple, … that's all."

"You did well," the doctor stated before making a notation on the chart and turning back to Rodger. "Try to remember the words apple, book, hammer, because in a few minutes I'm going to ask you to repeat them again. Can you tell me how old you are?"

"Seventy-six."

"Can you count backward from 100 by sevens, like this, 100, 93, 86?

"100, 93 … That's enough."

The doctor made another notation in the chart before asking him to repeat the three words he'd recited earlier.

"Three words?"

"Yes. Can you remember what they were?"

"Apple was one, and I think hammer."

"Can you remember the other one?

"No."

"That's okay, you're doing fine."

Rodger beamed with pride as the doctor made another note in the chart. Next, he handed him a piece of paper and a pencil and asked him to draw a clock.

I watched as he drew a shaky, lopsided circle and began placing the numbers one through twelve on the clock face. He remembered most of the numbers, but the placement was off. Instead of putting them evenly around the circle, his numbers marched up the left side of the drawing only.

That's not good, I thought, carefully scanning the doctor's face for a clue to his thoughts.

After adding a few more notes to the chart, the doctor turned to me. "It's about what we expected. He shows signs of moderate cognitive impairment. It's an indication of onset age-related dementia. We're going to want to monitor him to see if it progresses. I understand he lives with you and your husband, is that still correct?"

"Yes. I stay at home with him while Mike goes to work."

"I can take care of myself but she won't let me. It's too much for her," Rodger added firmly.

"What does this mean as far as his care goes?" I asked. "He's already on a lot of medication. I worry about adding to that stew and creating more problems with unexpected side effects. I've learned over the years that his reactions to medications are often the opposite of what we expect."

"At this stage there's no need for medication. I'll just see him every three months and keep an eye on him. It's not usual for people his age to have some impairment, and with his medical history it's a wonder he's doing as well as he is. You're doing a great job with him. He's lucky to have you."

"She's all right. She worries too much. I remember everything. I remember in Pittsburgh I didn't have so many doctors. I'm tired and sick of coming here."

The doctor placed his hand on my shoulder in a gesture of support and eased us out the door with a promise that I'd receive a letter in the mail informing us of his next appointment.

"Why do I have to go to the doctor so much? All they do is bullshit the time away. Remember words, draw something. I know where I live. It's bullshit."

Despite the ruckus it caused the night before, I pictured myself on the couch with my feet up watching *Dr. Phil*, sipping a chilled glass of wine once we got home. He'd be exhausted by the time we arrived and ready for a nap before dinner.

As delightful as that sounded, I pushed the image from my mind. I refuse to use alcohol as a crutch. If I felt I needed a drink the night before, I wouldn't have gone anywhere near it. I couldn't afford to be weak when others around me were falling apart. I'd learned that lesson living with an alcoholic for so many years. Booze does not alleviate problems, it makes them worse. Despite my efforts, my father-in-law was falling apart, piece by piece. I had to keep my wits about me if I had any hope of saving him from himself.

Over the next several months we witnessed a slow yet steady decline in Rodger's health. He went from seeing his doctor every three months to going in almost monthly. There were recurring bouts of bronchitis and pneumonia, requiring admission to the hospital for several days. I sat at his bedside from early morning until late in the evening each time, making sure his medication was crushed and mixed with applesauce, and he wasn't given the laxatives he'd insist he needed every time a new hospital worker entered his room. It didn't matter if it was a doctor or a maintenance person, no one got away without hearing about his bowel movements in great detail. Unfortunately, with multiple shift changes and personnel rotations, he always found someone who would comply with his request and bring him a laxative when I stepped out for a break or went home for the night. Then someone would add a note to his chart, requesting that he be given a prescription when it was time to leave the hospital. The weeks following an admission were always difficult. His routine had been disrupted, he was given food he wasn't supposed to eat, and he'd be furious with me when his laxatives were taken away. A three-day hospital stay could result in three weeks of drama at home. Each night I prayed he would remain healthy long enough to regain his strength before the next bout of illness struck. He was losing weight with each admission, and he wasn't anywhere near as strong as he had been just a few months ago. I also prayed for the wisdom and guidance to always do what was best for him. Some nights I prayed so hard and so long I wondered if God was tired of hearing from me and turned away in order to help some other less-demanding soul. I certainly hoped not, for without God's help I'd never get it right.

Chapter 15

Three weeks had passed since Rodger had come home from his latest trip to the hospital, and I was sitting in the family room watching a gentle snowfall cover the trees in the backyard. Although I dislike the cold, I love to see snow in the winter. It reminds me of my childhood in New York, at a time when kids were sent outdoors to play regardless of the weather, and the only way to stay warm was to keep moving. I smiled at the thought of endless sled runs down Dead Man's Hill and skating on the frozen creek down the road. Sometimes our neighbor across the street would flood the field next to his house and invite all the neighborhood kids over to skate. It was safer than the creek, and the moms liked it, but it was small, making racing impossible. And there was always the danger of tripping on one of the small clumps of grass that managed to poke through the ice. I had fallen many times, scraping my hands or chin on the uneven surface. Despite the tiny scar on my chin, I remember those days with great fondness. The snowmen we built were amazing, if only in our own minds, decked out as they were with castoff clothes donated by parents thrilled to get the kids out of their hair for a while. And, finally, when everyone was nearly too frozen to move anymore, someone's mother would call us in for hot cocoa, each cup adorned with a bobbing, full-size marshmallow. If we were very lucky, she'd also serve some still-warm-from-the-oven Toll House cookies, chock-full of chocolate chips.

Maybe later I'll invite Rodger to go out and build a snowman with me, I thought. *The fresh air will do him good, and if I can persuade Mike to join us, he can do the heavy lifting. When we're done, I'll make a pot of hot chocolate and open the bag of Oreos stashed in the pantry.*

Just as I was about to call the men and ask them to go out and play, I noticed Rodger trying to go upstairs. He was having trouble lifting his leg high enough to place his foot on the first step. Not quite understanding what I was seeing, I didn't go to his aid immediately. After another try, he was able to get up the first and second steps. He had a little difficulty with the third and fourth steps but recovered quickly and made it to the landing between the first and second flights without any trouble. It was when he tried to scale the second, steeper set of stairs that I realized he was in serious danger. He grasped the railing with both hands and was trying hard to lift one foot then the other to no avail. If he got partway up those stairs and lost his footing, he could end up seriously hurt.

"Don't move!" I shouted. "Stay right where you are!"

"What's wrong?" Mike called out and rushed out of the home office where he was busy paying bills.

"Rodger, don't move. I'm coming to help you," I shouted again, ignoring Mike for the moment. True to form, Rodger ignored me. To him, being told not to move appeared to mean go as fast as you can before she catches you.

He'd made it almost to the top step before I was able to reach him, but the effort had sapped his strength. That and whatever was wrong with him made it impossible for him to get his foot up over the last step and onto the floor above. He was teetering back and forth, ready to fall, when I finally reached him. Knowing that if he did fall he'd take me down with him, I placed both hands in the middle of his back and pushed. The momentum got him up the last stair and a half step more before he fell gently to his knees on the carpet. I moved up beside him and offered my hand to help him up just as Mike joined me and lifted him to his feet.

"What happened?" Mike asked, the worry lines on his forehead more pronounced than ever.

"She pushed me!" Rodger gasped. "She's trying to kill me."

"I pushed you because I was trying to save you. You almost fell down the stairs." I felt tears of anger and frustration gathering in my eyes.

Here we go again, I thought. *I try to save him and he accuses me of hurting him. I've had just about enough of this bullshit!"*

"You saw her, don't deny it!" Rodger shouted at Mike.

"I did see her," Mike said in a voice as calm and low as he could make it under the circumstances. "She did it so you wouldn't fall backward down the stairs. She saved you."

"I don't need her to save me. I can walk on my own. She's crazy."

"What's wrong with your legs?" I asked trying to remain calm and redirect his line of thinking.

"Nothing. Nothing's wrong with my legs. When you're old you have trouble sometimes. That's all. Get away from me. You tried to kill me. I don't trust you."

I lost it then. "It doesn't make sense to push someone UP the stairs if you're trying to kill them. If you want to hurt someone, you push them DOWN the stairs, and you don't stand behind them so if they do fall, you fall too. I'm sick and tired of your bullshit. All day, every day, I do everything I can to help you. I take you to the doctor, and I make sure you get your medicine. I cook for you. I feed you when you're sick, and I sit at your bedside for hours, day after day when you're in the hospital, to make sure you get good care. I work my ass off trying to do what's best for you, and you fight me every step of the way. What the hell is wrong with you?"

"Nothing. Nothing is wrong with me. See, she's crazy," he shouted at Mike. "Tell her I can take care of myself. I don't need anything from her."

"Yes you do!" Mike shouted back. "Without her, you wouldn't have survived this long."

"Ah, you believe everything she says. You don't listen to me. She tried to kill me and you do nothing. I'm going to tell the doctor."

"Do you want me to dial the number for you?" I asked, still bristling with anger.

"No! I'm going to my room. You stay away from me."

"Gladly!" I stormed down the stairs with Mike right behind me.

"I can't believe I just did that," I said to Mike, after taking a few moments to get my emotions under control.

"Did what?" Mike asked.

"Hollered at him that way. I demanded to know what's wrong with him when I know full well what his problems are. What I really need to know is what the hell is wrong with me. Why do I let him get to me that way? Why do I expect rational thought from someone who can't think straight most of the time? I try and try to keep the anger from bubbling up, but sometimes it gets away from me. I hate that I'm so weak. I'm not the person I thought I was when we started this."

"And who was that?"

"A good person. A caring person. Someone who would provide the best possible care for a family member I love, even when it's not easy. I knew it would be hard sometimes, but I had no idea it would be like this and I'd make such a mess of things. There I was, sitting on the loveseat watching the snow, about to invite the two of you outside to build a snowman with me, when everything turned to shit in a moment because I tried to save him from falling down the stairs."

"What exactly happened? I heard you call out to him and rushed to see what was wrong but the only part I saw was him teetering at the top of the steps, about take both of you down. I was terrified you'd both fall before I could get to you. Thank God you pushed him when you did."

"Too bad he doesn't see it that way," I answered softly. "And too bad I didn't handle it better when he didn't."

"You didn't do anything wrong. When he gets like that, he won't listen to reason and often the only way to get through to him is to shout back. The doctors have told you that, the people from the mental health clinic have told you that, and I tell you that. You are a good person and somewhere deep inside he knows it."

"I hope so," I said, wishing that deep inside I could believe it as well.

I tossed and turned throughout the night, struggling with guilt and self-doubt. I tried so hard to remain calm when he acted out.

Shame coursed through me each time I felt my pulse race and my face get hot, sure signs of anger beginning to build. I fought valiantly to rein in any negative thoughts and repeatedly reminded myself that he's sick.

Please help me to do better, I prayed. *The very actions that set me off are why needs me. Who else would put up with him? Even when he's not delusional, he's self-centered and rude. He has the manners of a wildebeest, and the arrogance of a Donald Trump.*

I couldn't help but giggle at that last characterization, accurate as it might be. I closed my eyes and pictured a weak and elderly wildebeest with a bad comb-over demanding to know why I had pushed him. Vowing to do better next time, I closed my eyes and tried again to get some rest. I was going to need it if what had just happened meant what I was convinced it did. His routine was about to change again and, with it, more restrictions in his movements that required even more monitoring. My latest determination to be a better person and a better caregiver were about to be tested—again.

Dear Lord, hold me in your love and light. Show me what to do and provide the resources to do what is best for him, despite my weaknesses.

As the sound of Rodger's steady snores assured me that he was in no danger at the moment, I quietly cried myself to sleep

Chapter 16

Three weeks later, after a visit to his primary care doctor to verify the need for another evaluation, Rodger and I were again sitting in the neurologist's office. I was very apprehensive and hoping he wouldn't dismiss, as he had before, my concerns about the possibility that Rodger's shaking hands and odd movements were signs of Parkinson's disease.

"Mr. Carducci, you're back. What brings you here today?"

"She worries too much. Sometimes when you're old, you shake."

The doctor didn't answer. Instead he directed his attention to his computer screen for several minutes. I hoped he was reading the notes from the primary care doctor who made the referral and not contemplating his next move on a video game.

"Tell me what's been happening lately," he said, looking to me this time.

After I told him about the incident on the stairs, in detail, the doctor asked Rodger to stand up, then return to his seat. Next he asked him to walk toward the door and turn around and come back.

"Hmm," he said.

I knew that was doctor code for, "I'm thinking of something I'm not quite ready to share yet."

"Can you smile for me?" the doctor asked him.

I'd like to see that too, I thought. Rodger rarely smiled, but when he did, it transformed his face and I could see hints of the handsome young man he once was.

"You do have Parkinson's disease," the doctor gently told Rodger.

"My sister has Parkinson's disease," was his only reply.

"How can you tell he has it now when you were so sure he didn't have it when I first brought him to see you?"

"In addition to the hand tremors, he now has difficulty moving from a seated to standing position, and his balance is off. He has to take many small steps to turn around, and he shows clear signs of facial masking, or difficulty using the muscles in his face to smile or show emotion. His arms hang straight down when he walks. They don't swing like they do for you and me. All are clear indications of Parkinson's disease."

Most of which he also exhibited on our first visit, I thought but didn't say.

The doctor went on to explain that there are two forms of Parkinson's disease. One is systemic and the other is caused by long-term use of some drugs, including many of those Rodger took for his schizophrenia before safer, more effective drugs came into use. Roger could have developed either form. Since there was a family history of Parkinson's disease, he'd be at risk for that—and the form caused by long-term use of some medications. The problem was, he explained, there wasn't a test to determine which form he had.

"The only way we'll know is by how he reacts to the medication I'm going to start with. If the symptoms don't abate, it was caused by the drugs he was given and there's nothing we can do."

"What happens if he has that type?"

"The symptoms will worsen over time, affecting more and more muscles until he's unable to move on his own."

A horrible thought occurred to me. The heart is a muscle and it takes muscles to breath. If the medication failed to work, Rodger had just been condemned to a slow and painful death.

Seeming to sense my thoughts, the doctor said, "Let's not assume the worst. Pick up the prescription on the way out and make sure he takes it every day. I'll see him again in a month. We'll know then what we're dealing with and how to plan for his future.

"My sister has Parkinson's disease, and Michael J. Fox has it too," Rodger pronounced before turning to leave. "They still live. You can live a long time with Parkinson's disease. I told you she worries too much."

When we went back for a follow-up visit a month later, I was happy to report that within a few days of taking the new medication, Rodger had improved a great deal. He was walking better and he no longer looked so stern all the time.

"I'm glad to hear that," the doctor answered. "I advise you to limit his use of stairs as much as possible. At his age a fall would be devastating. Other than that, keep doing what you're doing and bring him in to see me every three months. If he seems to be getting worse, call for another appointment. If the change is sudden and drastic, get him to an emergency room right away.

"You're a lucky man, Mr. Carducci. Your daughter-in-law takes good care of you."

To my surprise, Rodger nodded in agreement and said, "Without her, I'd be a goner. She's my best friend."

Later that night, when I reported what the doctor said and Rodger's unexpected response, Mike and I wondered where that had come from.

"See, I told you that somewhere deep inside he knows you're looking out for him, and he appreciates it more than you know. And so do I."

Chapter 17

Rodger improved a lot on the new medication. He enjoyed going for walks again, although he didn't walk as far or as long as he had in the past. I kept a close eye on the amount of time he was out of my sight, fearing that one day his dementia would cause him to forget where he lived. It may have been a concern for him as well, but I knew he'd never admit it. He no longer took long looping walks through the neighborhood and returned home to report on the new home construction going on in the growing development, and he spent a lot more time sitting on the bench out front, watching the birds fly in for a snack, or listening to them sing a tune of thanks after having eaten their fill.

One afternoon I was surprised to hear him come in within minutes of heading out.

"What brings you back so soon?" I asked.

"Nothing brings me back. I walked back," he snapped.

He avoided looking me in the eye and went directly to his room. I listened to him pacing, hoping he'd calm himself and come out and tell me what was bothering him. When he was still doing it a full half hour later, I feared he'd fret himself into a meltdown. Deciding to try and avoid a difficult time for both of us, I climbed the stairs and gently knocked on his door.

"Come in," he responded.

I found him seated on the couch. He was gasping for air and his hair was mussed, a clear sign he had been running his hands through it as he paced.

"Did something happen to you on your walk? Did one of the big dogs bark at you?"

"No. The dogs are inside a fence. They don't bother me."

"Then why did you come back from your walk so soon? Do you feel sick?"

"No."

"Rodger, please tell me what's wrong. I heard you pacing up here. I know you're worried about something. Maybe I can help."

"Nobody can help. Everybody has to die sometime. You're born with a destiny. My mother always said, 'You're born, you suffer, you die.'"

"It's true we all die sometime, and we have to deal with hard things in life, but there's joy and beauty too. So I hope you stick around for a long time. Now what's on your mind today?"

After a long silence, he finally began to speak. "I had a spell when I was walking. My feet wouldn't move. I think I'm going to die soon. I can't go for a walk anymore. I had a spell in Pittsburgh, and Shirley told me I'd die before her. She was wrong. She died first. It was her destiny."

My heart nearly broke as I realized how frightened he must have been.

"I think I know what happened, but just to be sure I'm going to check your temperature and heart rate and listen to your lungs. Okay?"

"Do what you want. Everyone has a destiny. You can't deny it."

"Everything looks good," I reported after doing all the things I had mentioned and checked his blood pressure as well. His BP was elevated a bit, probably due to his fear, so I wasn't concerned. I'd check it again in an hour to be sure, but I was confident he was in no danger.

"Do you remember the doctor telling you that you have Parkinson's disease?"

"I remember."

"Well, sometimes people with Parkinson's disease have trouble walking. Do you remember when you had a hard time lifting your feet to go up the steps?"

"I remember. You pushed me. But you didn't try to kill me," he answered.

I swear I saw a glimpse of humor in his eye when he said the last few words.

"That's right. I didn't try to kill you," I smiled at him. "I'll call the neurologist and tell him what happened. He may want to change the dosage of your medicine. You just started taking it, so it may take some time to figure out how much you should be taking."

A quick call to the doctor confirmed what I suspected. It was the Parkinson's disease that had caused his brief problem. The doctor told me that he'd most likely continue to have some symptoms, even on the medication, and reminded me that we were dealing with a progressive disease. He was doing well now, and there was no need to jump in and change things yet.

I reported what the doctor said, as close to word for word as I could. I realized he was looking at me closely and suspected he was looking for signs that I wasn't telling the truth. I'd never lie to him or hide anything from him, but I also knew I wouldn't convince him of that. It wasn't in him to really trust anyone. I simply patted his hand and asked that he promise to tell me if anything like that happened again. He said he would and declared he was tired and needed to rest, so I gave him a quick kiss on the cheek and left the room.

After several days passed without a recurrence of any problems, Mike and I felt it would be okay to go out for a while. It had become a weekly habit to attend 5:00 p.m. Mass and then have dinner at a local restaurant. Not exactly a raucous date night, but we had come to rely on the time away from home together to relax and enjoy one another's company. I always prepared Rodger's dinner and left the plate on the table for him to heat in the microwave when he was ready to eat. I suspected he enjoyed having time alone as much as we did. The evening had gone very well, and I was comfortably full and a little bit sleepy when we pulled into the garage. I thought about inviting Mike to spend some time in the hot tub later. We could sit in the bubbling water and look at the stars while any remaining tension swirled away and disappeared into the filter. I could feel my shoulders relaxing just thinking about it. Sometimes they rose so high with tension I thought they would touch my ears.

I knew that wasn't going to happen the moment I opened the door and saw the full plate of food still sitting on the table.

"Something's very wrong," I said to Mike when he followed me in.

He knew immediately that I was right when he saw where I was pointing. His father would never willingly miss a meal.

"Dad, are you okay?" he called as he turned and bolted up the steps.

I followed close behind. We froze when we saw what awaited us at the top of the stairs. Rodger's body lay in the hallway between his room and the bathroom. Pain and infinite regret engulfed me at the thought that he had died alone after I had reassured him it wasn't his time. Had the doctor or I missed something? And my poor husband, the agony he must be feeling. I was fighting back tears, bracing for the difficult time ahead when Rodger suddenly sat up and spoke.

"What's up?" he asked.

"What do you mean, what's up?" Mike shook his head in confusion. "What happened? What are you doing on the floor?"

I was as dumbfounded as Mike. I tried to take in the surreal scene in front of me. Goosebumps raised the hair on my arms, and my heart rate was going through the roof. Relief mixed with panic. Relief that he was alive and seemingly okay; panic that I might be imagining things. Was he dead and I couldn't accept it? Was I seeing things?

"Dad, what are you doing? Let me help you up," Mike said. His voice sounded as strained as mine would have if I had tried to speak at that moment. Luckily, all I had to do was listen.

"I thought I was having a heart attack, so I lay down so I wouldn't hurt myself when I died."

I shook my head at the implied, "Duh!" in his voice, as if we were dimwits for not realizing the logic behind his actions. While I tried to process what I was hearing, Mike led his father into his sitting room. I followed and joined them on the sofa.

"What made you think you were having a heart attack?" Mike

asked. "Were you having chest pains?"

"No chest pains," he answered.

"Is anything hurting you?" I asked, placing my fingers on his wrist to check his pulse.

It was a little fast but strong and regular enough to reassure me. I cast Mike a look of relief and waited for Rodger to continue.

"I went down to eat and I felt weak. I had a hard time standing up. I thought I was going to have a heart attack, so I came up here and lay down so I didn't hurt myself when I died."

"Do you feel weak now?" I was baffled by his reasoning, but I wasn't going to address that until I checked him out some more.

"No, I don't feel weak. I'm okay now. Don't worry about me."

"I want you to sit here and don't move until I listen to your heart and check your blood pressure. If there's any sign that there's anything wrong, we'll call an ambulance and get you to a hospital."

Just as had happened a few days before, his vital signs were within normal range.

"There are no signs of heart trouble," I assured both father and son. "Rodger, listen to me," I said calmly. "What happened to you was not a heart attack. You felt weak because of the Parkinson's disease. I'm convinced you're fine now, but if you're worried we'll take you to the hospital."

"No. I don't want to go to the hospital. I'm okay. I didn't die. You worry too much. What's for supper? I gotta eat sometime."

"I'm sure you're hungry," I said. "It's way past your suppertime. I'll heat it up and bring it to you."

"I can fix it myself," he answered.

"I'll get it and bring it on a tray. You sit here with Mike and I'll be right back."

I left the room before he had a chance to object again. After delivering his meal, I left the two of them alone to talk. Mike needed some time with his father after the trauma of thinking he'd lost him, and I needed time to figure out how I was going to explain to Mike that our date nights were over, and his father could never be left alone again, not even for short periods of time. What I didn't realize, until he shared his thoughts later, was that Mike had instantly come to the same conclusion. He told me that he wondered how much more I could take, and how could he ask it of me. I was suffering in order to take care of his father, and he had to do something to take some of the pressure off. The time may have come to make other arrangements for his care.

"No. I can't do it. He'll die within weeks if we put him in long-term care," I insisted when Mike spoke of admitting him. "You know how he is. He'll tell the nurses to go away and take care of the sick people, insisting he can take care of himself. Before long he'll start cheeking his medication and have a psychotic break. If that doesn't destroy him, he'll get an infection or pneumonia that will go unnoticed until it's too late. He'll die of neglect, not because the hospital staff is uncaring or negligent, but because they have so many patients who demand their attention while he's insisting he's fine. I couldn't live with myself if I let that happen, and neither could you."

"All that may be true, but what about you? Aren't you denying the truth when you say you're fine? Aren't you putting your health at risk by insisting his needs come first?"

"I don't know what you're talking about," I insisted.

"Oh please! What about the long days and nights you spend at his bedside whenever he's in the hospital, and the sleepless nights you spend worrying about him when he's home. It's all taking more of a toll on you than you realize. Just the everyday routine of seeing to it that he takes his ever-growing number of medications and breathing treatments on time, making his meals, and getting him to bathe and brush his teeth must be exhausting. When you add in scheduling and getting him to his many doctor visits, or making sure he doesn't wander off or accidentally hurt himself, you barely have time to take a breath. You're constantly monitoring how he looks, talks, and moves. You can't go on like this. I'm as concerned about you as I am for him."

I had to admit he was right. But I couldn't help hovering over Rodger, looking for any slight change signaling another bout of bronchitis or pneumonia. I looked for changes in his behavior that would indicate an increase in paranoia or delusions. I rarely slept through the night anymore, leaving me tired and out of sorts with both men in my life.

"I know I need a break, but how can I go away? Who will care for Rodger?

"I've been thinking about that," Mike answered. "I remember the social worker telling us the VA hospital offers respite care for people like us. With his 100% service-related disability designation, he qualifies. We can look into it and find out how to get you some rest before you collapse. You need it. We both need it."

"All right, I'll call the patient advocate in the morning and ask about the service. I think I remember someone saying we can admit him to the hospital for thirty days of respite care a year, but for no more than fourteen days at a time."

"That sounds right," Mike said. "Imagine two weeks away, just the two of us, with no schedules to meet and no need to get out of bed until we're ready."

"I'll make the call first thing in the morning."

The idea of going on vacation was exciting, but I wasn't getting my hopes up yet. The offer of respite care seemed too good to be true.

Chapter 18

"Ready to go?" Mike asked.

"More than ready," I said.

I couldn't believe we were actually going to Hawaii for twelve days. When I called the patient advocate, I expected to be told we had either misunderstood, or that respite care was no longer available. Happily, that was not the case. It took time to work out the logistics, but after filling out the required forms, waiting for approval, and praying a bed would be available on the dates we needed, it worked out.

I tried to relax as we headed to the airport, but I kept thinking about how I almost backed out that morning when I saw the room waiting for him. I knew he was being admitted to the hospital nursing home wing, but I wasn't been prepared for what that meant—and from Rodger's reaction, neither was he. Some patients were walking the halls, others sat in wheelchairs, seemingly oblivious to anything going on around them. TVs blared, and the noise level was already making him nervous. On top of that, he'd be sharing a room with a man who had obviously been there a long time. Family pictures and cards, yellowing with age, were displayed on the walls and windowsill. The closet they were to share was full, leaving only a shelf for Rodger's clothes. I knew it wouldn't hold the two weeks' worth of clothing, pajamas, and the few personal items I packed for him. But what that bothered me most was the door leading directly outside located only a few steps from the room. There was no way the hospital staff could see it from the nurses' station. Rodger wouldn't hesitate to make a quick exit if he decided it was time to go for walk. Lord only knew how long he'd be gone before anyone missed him. Seeing that, I knew I had to remind them he was at risk for wandering. I had put that on his preadmission questionnaire, but there was a good chance the information hadn't made it into his chart.

Upon hearing my concerns, the nurse said, "Don't leave," and picked up the phone. After speaking softly to whoever was on the other end and making a note on a slip of paper, she turned to me and said, "I'm sorry to tell you this, but you're going to have to move his things to the fourth floor. He can't stay here."

I smiled with relief. The doctors and nurses up there knew and liked Rodger, and patients likely to wander were fitted with a bracelet that automatically locked the exits when they approached. He would be safe.

"What are you thinking about?" Mike asked.

"How glad I am we can get away for a while and ..."

"And?"

"And I hope he'll be okay."

"He will be. And just to be sure, we can call the nurses' station to check on him while we're away. But please, promise you'll stop worrying long enough to have a good time with me."

"I promise."

I pushed aside my misgivings about leaving and what we'd face when we got home, and imagined walking on warm sand in the moonlight, holding hands with Mike. I could almost hear the sound of the surf mingling with the gentle notes of Hawaiian music, and feel his lips, soft and warm, on mine.

We spent the first two days doing as little as possible. We slept late and had a light breakfast of fresh fruit. In the afternoon we lay on the beach, dividing the time between reading and dozing. On the afternoon of the second day the warm sun worked its magic and muscles, long tense from fatigue and stress, released their grip. Slowly my worries began to fade into the background. *I will take advantage of this respite. I will laugh and swim and dance and enjoy every moment with my loving husband.*

"Thank you," I said, when I looked over and noticed Mike studying me.

"For what?"

"For loving me. For knowing how much I needed this. For being as special as you are."

"You're amazing," he said. His eyes filled with unshed tears. He reached across the narrow span of sand separating us and took my hand in his. "All I did was make arrangements for this vacation. You do the hard stuff every day. I feel so bad for you, having to deal with him every day."

"Don't feel bad for me. It's not easy for you either. I admit it's a lot harder than I thought it would be, but I do it because I love him and I love you. Family takes care of family, and we're in this together. And I do thank you for this vacation, more than you know. Let's make a pact to get away more often. It doesn't have to be two weeks in Hawaii. It can be as simple as a long weekend at home alone once in a while."

"You have a deal," Mike readily agreed. "I hope you remember this conversation when we're back home and things are getting tough again."

Once we were rested, we ventured out to have fun. We went to a *luau*, savoring the sweet and salty taste of roast pig and the odd tang of poi. I loved the catamaran rides, with the rocking of the waves and the feel of the seaspray on my skin. One of the guides told of coming to Hawaii on vacation and never leaving. He used all his savings to purchase the catamaran and now spent his days on the water, often taking it out early in the morning and diving for lobster for his breakfast. We went sea kayaking and swam with giant sea turtles.

One of my favorites was the day we went to a working ranch for a two-hour horseback ride. The guides led us across the beach and up a winding mountain trail. One moment we were surrounded by trees and grass, enjoying the shade and listening to exotic birdcalls, and the next the trail widened, allowing us to stop and rest the horses for a bit. Immediately people began to take pictures.

Spread before us was a view I'll never forget. The sky was so vividly blue it almost hurt to look at it. Fluffy white clouds drifted over the ocean, crystalline blue close to shore then fading to black as the ocean deepened. Framing it all was a double rainbow. *It's going to be okay,* a voice whispered in my soul. *I am with you even when you can't hear me.*

I made the sign of the cross and silently thanked God for the blessings in my life. And, yes, my father-in-law, as difficult as he could be, was one of them. We called the hospital every other day to check on him, and the nurses assured us everything was going well. Rodger always said the same thing when he spoke to either of us.

"Hi. How's everything? Don't worry about me. I was in the hospital a long time. I know what to do. I'll stay here if they let me."

Each time we reminded him that we'd be there in a few days to take him home. He seemed to forget what the patient advocate, his doctor, the admitting nurse, and I had tried to make clear to him. Respite care is only for a few days. If someone didn't come and take him home at the end of that time, the hospital would move him to a private nursing home, and the family would be responsible for the cost of moving him and any fees for his stay. The mention of having to pay would be enough to quiet him on the subject for a few minutes, but I knew he'd say the same thing the next time we called.

On our last day of vacation I rose early to sit on the balcony and watch the sunrise. As the morning mist began to clear, so did my thoughts about going home. As appealing as the idea of diving for lobsters for breakfast and riding a catamaran every day might be for some, it was not the life I wanted. I was rested and ready to go back.

Just as I was about to go in and get ready for the day, an odd feeling swept over me. I was aware that something was happening to me, but I couldn't define what it was. My senses were muted. Sounds faded, and my body felt slow and heavy. *This is not good,* I thought.

The left side of my neck began to tingle. The hair on my arms stood straight up. The feeling moved down my left arm, eventually affecting my entire left side. I wasn't able to move or call out for help.

"I'm having a stroke!"

I prayed for Mike and my kids, dreading the burden caring for me would put on them if I lived. Although no tears fell, I wept inside for the grief they would feel if I died. *What will become of Rodger?* Almost as soon as I completed that thought, the tingling went away. The sense of heaviness lifted and I was able to move.

"What was that?" I said out loud, testing my voice.

It sounded perfectly normal. In fact, everything had gone back to normal. Despite the fear I felt when it was happening, I convinced myself it was nothing. There was no need to mention it to anyone. I'm strong and healthy. The tingle and goose bumps must have been caused by a wayward breeze coming off the ocean. Yes, that was it. It was time to go in and get ready for one final adventure before going home.

I put a smile on my face and went to wake Mike. From the moment he arrived in Hawaii, he'd been looking forward to fulfilling a long-delayed wish. He was going to go surfing for the first time. I'd have tried it too, but I knew I wouldn't be able to get up on the board. My creaky knees would never cooperate.

"You did it! Hurray!" I cheered for Mike the first time he caught a wave.

He smiled proudly before turning back into the surf for another ride. Clearly he loved every minute of it, even when he fell off the board or was upstaged by a six-year-old who made it look easy from the first try. I was delighted to see him having such a good time. My heart swelled with love. To have this wonderful man in my life is a blessing I will treasure always.

Chapter 19

When I got to the hospital to take Rodger home, I was shocked to find a sign on the door to his room announcing the patient was in isolation and all visitors were to don a yellow gown and gloves before entering.

"What's going on with Mr. Carducci?" I asked the nurse manning the station right outside his room.

"And who are you?" she responded.

I explained who I was, that I was there to take him home from respite care, and repeated my question. I tried to hide the anger I was feeling at not having been told he was ill when I called to let them know when I'd be there to pick him up.

"Your father-in-law has MRSA, and precautions have to be taken to keep him from infecting others."

"What's that? How serious is it? When did he get it? How did he get it?"

Seeing my distress, the nurse set aside the chart she was working on and explained. "MRSA stands for Methicillin-resistant Staphylococcus aureus. It's a staph germ that does not get better with antibiotics that usually cure staph infections. People who spend a lot of time in the hospital are at risk of catching it. It can be very dangerous to those with compromised immune systems."

"So he got it here?"

"We don't know for sure when or where he got it. Hospital policy is to test all patients being admitted these days. Your father-in-law has a MRSA colonization in his nasal passages. That's the reason for the isolation room and the gowns and gloves for visitors. He doesn't have an active MRSA infection now. However, it's possible for him to infect others if he puts his fingers in his nose then touches common surfaces."

"Does that mean he can't go home? Are my husband and I at risk? He lives with us. I take care of him every day."

"Oh, he can go home. In fact, he's all packed and ready to go. You're no more at risk now than you were before. However, if you do get an infection in a cut or sore, you need to tell your doctor about your exposure. You should be fine."

"So I can go in and collect his things?"

"Yes, but make sure you put on a gown and gloves before entering the room."

"Why? I'm just going to do what's necessary to get him checked out and take him home. It makes no sense to protect me here so I can be exposed 24/7." Before the nurse had a chance to answer, I said, "You don't have to say it. I know. It's hospital rules."

"What are you dressed up for?" Rodger asked when I entered his room. "You think you're a doctor now?"

The smirk on his face irritated me almost as much as the prospect of having to don gown and gloves to enter the room, grab his suitcase and prescriptions to be filled at the hospital pharmacy, take the gown and gloves off and dispose of them in the hospital waste container outside his room, stand in line for his medication, take it and the suitcase to the car, and put on gown and gloves again in order to go back in and get him to take him home.

I swallowed my feelings and smiled at him. "I look kind of silly, don't I? But the doctor said I have to wear this in your room. Are you ready to go?"

"I've been ready," he answered. "They won't let me stay here."

"That's good. Your home is with us. We missed you when we were away."

"Yeah, you missed me. You must love me."

"We do," I said.

I also noticed he didn't return the sentiment.

We were both quiet on the drive home. I kept glancing over at him, looking for signs that he'd managed to avoid taking his medication. At first I saw nothing and was silently thanking the hospital staff for their vigilance. It was when I was pulling into the driveway that I saw the subtle, involuntary movement of his head that indicated he had missed at least a few doses of his Zyprexa.

"Home sweet home," he said, as the rising garage door rattled up in welcome.

"Home sweet home," I agreed.

My vacation was definitely over.

The next several weeks were hectic. Rodger challenged me every chance he got. He didn't want to take so many pills. He needed laxatives. He knew how to cook. In the old country women didn't tell men what to do. Alone in his room during the day he paced and muttered. At night he walked the halls, the squeaky floorboard outside my bedroom waking me each time he came near. I did my best to take it in stride. His routine had been disturbed, and he was doing his best to cope with what seemed to be the ever-changing expectations of those around him. I bit my tongue when he snapped at me, I left the room when he made it clear my presence was unwanted, and over time I eased us back into our normal routine.

When I noticed the increasing number of hairs in my brush each morning, I refused to acknowledge the real reason it was happening. Instead I changed my shampoo and conditioner and scheduled appointments for color touch-ups farther apart. I convinced myself that the two other instances of tingling and goose bumps that occurred at odd moments were caused by the air conditioning coming on.

"Take me to the hospital," Rodger yelled out from the top of the stairs.

"What's wrong?" I called up to him.

Mike, who was home at the time, joined me to hear the answer.

"I can't piss."

"What do you mean, you can't pee?" I said.

"Since when?" Mike added.

"Since now. I need a tube. I have to be able to piss."

Soon we were all in the car on the way to the emergency room.

"If he's asking for a tube in his penis, he must be in pain. That's not something any man would ask for unless he had no choice," Mike said.

I agreed. My father-in-law was more likely to hide symptoms than pretend they were worse. Once, he even denied pain after falling and breaking a rib. My concern was how long he'd had this problem before saying anything, and how sick he might be.

After arriving at the hospital and filling out the triage form and waiting to be seen by a nurse, Rodger was again admitted to the hospital and a catheter was put in place. He had a bladder infection and was running a low-grade fever. Mike sat with him while I spoke with the admitting doctor and the nurse who would be in charge of his care. I stressed the importance of making everyone aware of his special needs. Crush his medication and put it in applesauce. No laxatives. Everyone had to be aware that he suffered from mental illness and early dementia, and he might decide he didn't need to be there any longer and wander off. He was recently diagnosed with Parkinson 's disease, so he was at risk of falling.

"Don't worry, Mrs. Carducci. All this is in his chart and we'll take good care of him," the nurse assured me.

"I'm sure you will," I answered.

I hoped the woman couldn't tell I was lying through my teeth. I'd seen too many screw-ups by well-meaning hospital personnel to ever feel at ease in leaving him.

"I'll be back in the morning to see how he is and to talk to his doctor."

"No need to hurry," the nurse answered. "Take some time for yourself while you can. The nurse on duty will be able to bring you up to date if you aren't here when the doctor arrives."

I thanked her for her concern and went in to say goodbye to Rodger, knowing I'd arrive at the hospital early and stay late every day as long as he was there. I hoped his stay would be short this time. His birthday was in a week, and his brother was planning to come for a visit. I hadn't told Rodger about the little party I was planning for fear something would come up and his brother wouldn't come. I knew Rodger wouldn't admit his disappointment to anyone. Instead he'd pace and wander through the house at night.

After three days he was sent home, with the catheter still in place, instructions on how to care for it, and an appointment to see a urologist in two weeks. He'd be home for his birthday.

The day before his discharge I received a call from the hospital social worker asking me to meet with her and his nurse before taking Rodger home.

"It's nothing to be concerned about," she assured me. "In fact, what we have in mind is a program that we hope will help keep Rodger out of the hospital."

I told her I was all for that and agreed to arrive at the hospital an hour early. When I got there, the social worker, a male nurse I had never met, and the patient advocate were waiting for me. When they explained what they had in mind, I was thrilled. Rodger was entitled to participate in a new Telehealth program, and they hoped we'd agree to have him monitored from home.

"How does it work?"

"My name is Jackson," the nurse said before explaining that if we agreed to take part in the program, they would provide us with a minicomputer that would connect to our phone line.

"Every morning you'll take Rodger's blood pressure, heart rate, oxygen levels, and weight, using connections to the telehealth machine. The information will go directly into his chart and I'll read the results. If I see any changes that require attention, I'll contact you to discuss what to do to improve things. If you see any signs that he's getting sick, or that his medications aren't working, you'll contact me directly and, if needed, I'll consult with the doctor. The hope is that by catching changes early we'll avoid the need for so many hospital admissions."

"Sign us up," I said. "I'll take all the help you can offer."

Rodger surprised me by accepting the device right away. I was afraid it would set him off again about the government knowing everything about you, but it didn't. He must have been tired of going to the hospital all the time as well.

He had been home for four days and was coping well with the catheter when a situation arose that had me reaching for the phone to consult with Jackson for the first time.

"Bobbi!" Rodger called out, panic making his voice tremble.

I looked up from the shirt I was ironing. I couldn't believe what I was seeing. Rodger was standing halfway down the stairs, with his pants around his knees, pointing at his privates.

"Come look at this," he said.

Not sure what was going through his mind, I hesitated to go near. "Look at what?"

My penis. Come here and look at it." He moved down a step. How he did it without tripping over his pants, I didn't know.

"Stay there, I'm coming. Why are your pants down?"

"I need you to look at my penis. I think this thing is leaking."

"Your penis is leaking?"

"No, the tube is leaking."

Relief washed over me. This was a catheter problem, not a dementia-related inappropriate moment. I went to him and led him safely up the stairs and into the bathroom. I checked the catheter and didn't see anything wrong, but I didn't really know how to tell if it was positioned exactly right.

"It looks okay to me, but I'm going to call Jackson and ask him if he thinks I should take you to the emergency room and get it checked."

"Who's Jackson?"

"He's a nurse at the hospital. I call him if I need advice about taking care of you."

"Call him," he insisted. "He knows what's what."

When I placed the call to Jackson, I didn't realize I was starting a relationship with a caring nurse who would come to mean more to Rodger and me than either of us could ever imagine.

"As long as there's no blood or yellowish discharge and he's able to pee, he's fine. He probably pulled on it a bit. Gently push the tube in a little. That should stop the leaking—and remind him not to handle the tube."

I put on some gloves and did as he said, gingerly adjusting the tube while praying he'd be catheter-free soon. There was little chance he'd stop fiddling with it, and sooner or later he'd end up with an infection. But at least I had Jackson to consult with. Already he'd spared us a trip to the hospital. For the first time in a long time I felt someone at the hospital was listening to me. We all sighed with relief when there were no more problems with the catheter and several days later he was able to return to the urologist and have it removed.

Chapter 20

"Tanti aguri a te. Tanti aguri a te. Tanti aguri bellisimo, Pop Pop. Tanti aguri a te."

Rodger's smile lit up the room as his grandson sang "Happy Birthday" in Italian. "Wow! Where did you learn that?" he asked. "You sing like you're from Italy."

"Aunt Bobbi taught me," answered ten-year-old Vito.

It had taken a bit of prompting to get him to sing in front of the family, but now that the song was over you could see the pride in his eyes. It was a rare moment of affection shared between grandfather and grandson. They seldom saw one another, and when they did age and shyness made communication difficult for both.

"Your accent is good. Maybe you can learn to speak more Italian. I remember some. When you visit again, I can—" Rodger began.

"Let's have some of that cake," his brother interrupted, breaking the spell.

I bit my tongue to keep from asking the man why he couldn't remain quiet long enough to allow Rodger to connect with Vito. Was it so hard to see him enjoying himself for a change? Or was he upset that he was no longer the center of his brother's attention? Ever since Dominick had arrived, Rodger hadn't taken his eyes of his younger brother. He tried hard to engage him in conversation, despite his limited communication skills and lack of any real connection, other than their years growing up in Italy. Even then their lives were vastly different. Roger had been the responsible, studious one; his brother had been the outgoing and mischievous one.

"You have no idea what my brother was like back then," Dominick had told me more than once. "He was brilliant. He could do calculus in his head. He'd get so mad at me when I couldn't grasp algebra. His mind worked too fast for me. Whenever he tried to help, we'd both end up frustrated. He called me stupid. I called him worse under my breath. He wrote beautiful poetry and spoke several languages. And he was absolutely fearless when it came to resisting the German soldiers who wanted to conscript him. He was often an arrogant s.o.b. He was my big brother and I idolized him, but he had no time for me."

And now you have no time for him, I thought. I knew it must have been hard growing up with a big brother like that. Most little kids would take that kind of treatment personally. But they were no longer boys, and clearly much of Rodger's arrogance and impatience and manic drive that affected their relationship then were early symptoms of the schizophrenia that would devastate his mind and rob him of the gifts he once had. Whenever Dominick would say that seeing his brother so diminished was too hard for him to deal with and that was why he rarely visited, I wanted to shake him and remind him that, as hard as it was for him, it was far worse for Rodger.

When the fog of mental illness lifted for a moment, he was painfully aware of what he had lost and the toll his illness had taken on his family. Where was the patience Dominick once expected from his brilliant older brother? Where was the compassion for a man who risked his life as a teenager against a deadly enemy? Where was the love of family that he professed to live by? I knew which brother was weak and which one had more guts and grace than the other could ever dream of having. I bristled with anger, but on this day I was determined to swallow my emotions by choking them down with birthday cake, despite the fact that the too-sweet icing didn't begin to temper the bitter taste in my mouth.

As soon as the gifts were opened and the cake eaten, the guests began to take their leave. The first was Rodger's brother. I had hoped he'd stay a bit longer, but I wasn't surprised when he made a swift exit. Despite the fact I knew things would never change, I had hoped he'd stay longer on what could be one of Rodger's last birthdays. The sad part was that Rodger accepted his brother's behavior without question. He smiled and shook his hand as he was leaving.

"Don't worry about me," he said. "I can take care of myself."

He said the same words to his younger son when he left. Neither man replied. Perhaps they hadn't heard him in their haste to leave. Rodger appeared to be shrinking as he stood in the doorway watching them. I was filled with admiration for him at that moment. Despite how hard it must have been, he did everything he could to hide how sick he was and how much their visit meant to him. He had no idea how diminished he looked even as he struggled to stand tall and pretend everything was all right. The only people he fooled were himself and those who didn't want to see. I pretended not to notice the glitter of unshed tears in eyes when he turned away from the door.

"Would you like another piece of cake?" I asked, hoping he didn't see the tears forming in my eyes.

"No thank you. I'm going to take a nap now. Why did people bring me presents? I don't need anything."

"They bring presents because they love you and it's your birthday."

"Vito, he sings good," Rodger chuckled. "He sounds like he's from Italy. Happy Birthday" he sang. "He loves me, yeah."

The next morning, right after sitting up in bed, I felt another spell coming on. It was stronger than it had ever been, and the tingling moved all the way down my body to my feet.

Please, don't let me die, I prayed. *Don't let Rodger or Mike find me like this.* I fought against the feeling of helplessness as my heart began to race. I wanted to move, to call out for help, but I couldn't make my limbs or my voice respond.

Think! What can you do?

A voice that sounded a lot like my deceased mother's responded, "Remain calm. Whatever this is, panicking won't help."

Easy for you to say, I thought, praying my mother's spirit was there to help and not to escort me into the light.

"Don't talk back, and get to a doctor," the voice continued.

There was a touch of humor in the voice that time. I figured if the ghost of my mother was amused, I wasn't going to die yet. I took a few more calming breaths and the spell began to clear. When it was gone and I was able to move, I dropped to my knees and thanked God and my mother for watching over me. As soon as I had Rodger settled for the morning, I called my doctor. Upon hearing my symptoms, he referred me to a neurologist and told me to request to be seen as soon as possible. I wondered if he suspected, as I did, that I was having TIAs, or small strokes. I didn't want to let it show, but I was scared.

Chapter 21

It was hard to tell who was more nervous when Mike and I sat in the doctor's office on the morning of my appointment. He had bitten his fingernails down to the quick in the car and still couldn't keep his hands out of his mouth. His left leg was in constant motion, vibrating against my chair. Guilt washed over me for adding to his worries.

I could feel my blood pressure rising. I hoped I wouldn't have another spell while waiting to see the doctor then wondered why the thought bothered me. What better place could there be? I'd get immediate attention and know once and for all what was wrong with me. Adding to my concern was the fact that Rodger was home alone and I had no idea how long this appointment would take. We didn't tell him why we were going out for the morning and he didn't ask. He seemed pleased to know he'd be on his own for a while. Oblivious to how weak he was, he promised to stay in the house to keep it safe while we were away. I fixed a plate of food and left it for him, ready to be heated in the microwave at lunchtime. He could choose between fruit or pudding cups for a snack. His medication wouldn't be due until late in the afternoon. Surely I'd be home by then. Wouldn't I?

I was close to convincing myself that the doctor would take one look at me and call for an ambulance when a nurse opened the door to the examining area and called my name. Phase two of the patient-doctor dance had begun. Phase one is arriving on time to sit in the waiting room for thirty minutes or more. Phase two is feeling incredibly grateful to be invited into an examining room to wait for another ten to twenty minutes and pass the time staring at pictures of human organs and blood vessels with descriptions of the very bad things that can happen when they aren't working right. I was mesmerized by a graphic picture of a bulging brain aneurism. Was something like that pulsing inside me? Hearing a soft rattle nearby,

I turned to look at Mike, expecting to see his left leg bouncing up and down against the leg of a chair again.

"Not me," he said, pointing to my feet dangling off the side of the examining table.

Without realizing it, I was tapping my heels together and wringing my hands. I remembered what my mother's voice told me the day of my last spell.

Take a deep breath and remain calm.

"Yes, Mother," I whispered.

"What did you say?" Mike asked.

"Nothing, just trying to calm my nerves."

"I know what you mean. I wish the doctor would get in here."

We waited another ten minutes before the door opened and the doctor stepped in. Apologizing for the delay, he introduced himself to me and then to Mike.

"So," he said, turning his full attention to me, "how are you today?"

"I'll know better how to answer that after you tell me what you think is happening to me."

"Fair enough," he said. "First, tell me what's been going on and when it started."

I told him about the spells and how the last one involved more of my body and lasted longer than the others, then he took a long look at my chart. Next he did a series of tests to determine if there was any sign of weakness on my left side. He listened to my heart and looked into my eyes and all the other things doctors usually do. He mentioned my blood pressure was elevated but I already knew that.

"The good news is, I don't believe you're having TIAs, or small strokes. But something is going on and we need to find out what it is. I'm going to order an extensive series of tests that may seem scary but won't hurt a bit. In the meantime, if you experience one of these spells again, I want you to call an ambulance and get to the hospital as soon as possible. I suspect you're having some kind of seizure activity. Or it may turn out to be something called G.O.K.

"What's that?" I could see by the look on Mike's face that he didn't know what it was either.

"G.O.K.," the doctor answered, "is a term I use for God Only Knows. Sometimes the body does things that we can't explain."

"What should I hope for?"

"G.O.K."

I didn't like hearing that. I wanted to know exactly what was happening to me and why. If the doctor really thought it was nothing serious, he wouldn't tell me to call an ambulance if it happened again.

When the nurse asked us to take a seat in the waiting room while she made some calls, I was convinced the doctor was as worried as I was. By the time we were cleared to leave, I had appointments for an MRI, an MRA, and a CAT scan, and I was wearing a monitor that would keep track of my heart for a few days. The walk to the car was made in silence as Mike and I tried to process what was happening.

"It's going to be all right," I finally said, reaching for Mike's hand.

"Yes it is. It has to be. I couldn't stand it if anything happened to you."

Rodger had eaten his lunch, had a snack, and was sound asleep in front of the TV when we got home. Relieved that he had done so well, I pushed aside my worries and put a load of laundry into the washer and began planning what to make for dinner. Something simple, I decided, pulling a package of ground beef out of the freezer. Cheeseburgers and a salad. Comfort food with a side of healthy would do nicely. That and a drink. I filled a highball glass with ice, added a shot of whiskey, topped it off with Coke, and enjoyed my appetizer while waiting for the laundry to finish.

The tension of the day, and the relaxing effects of the whiskey, meant that after getting Rodger settled for the night I was barely able to keep my eyes open. I didn't protest when Mike urged me to go up to bed, saying he hoped the drink would allow me to get a peaceful night's sleep.

"I know you often lie awake, worrying about the care you give my father. I feel so guilty that you're the one carrying the bulk of the burden, but I don't know what more I can do. I have to go to work. We need the money. And you're a much better caregiver then I could ever be. I admire your almost uncanny ability to detect changes in Rodger that signal something is wrong. You ask questions I'd never think of asking, and demand answers from his doctors with assurance that earns their respect. Jackson told me many doctors asked if you're a nurse. In fact, that's what you've become. My father's nurse. The problem as I see it is that you're so emotionally involved with your patient, you view every setback or new symptom as a sign of failure. Why can't you see all the things you do right, and how much my dad and I love and appreciate you?

I was too tired to take it all in. I fell into a deep sleep soon after getting into bed, rousing only briefly when Mike joined me. I wanted to reach out to him, tell him not to worry, but before I had a chance to say anything I drifted off again. In the morning I felt better, stronger than I had in a quite a while. I would undergo the tests, follow any recommended treatments, and I'd be fine. Jackson would continue to help me get the best care for Rodger, and life would go on. The first thing on my agenda was another long, hot shower to ease the kinks from my neck and shoulders. That and a cup of tea, and I'd be ready to conquer the world.

Chapter 22

Three weeks passed without any spells, and I was feeling cautiously hopeful when I entered the doctors' office to get my test results. No one had called, urging me to get to a hospital right away, or arranged for any prescriptions to be picked up at the pharmacy. I tried to get Mike to go to work that day. He had deadlines looming and work backing up. I didn't want to be responsible for making things harder for him.

"I've been symptom-free all this time. I promise I'll call you as soon as I have the results."

He wouldn't hear of it. "We're in this together," he said. "In sickness and in health, remember?"

Having him by my side helped me stay calm on the way in. It was only when I entered the doctor's office that my nerves began to get the best of me.

What if the news is really bad? It's going to be bad, I know it. A nurse would have called with good news. That's what they usually do. I'm going to go through that door and hear the words, "I'm so sorry, Mrs. Carducci, but there's nothing we can do."

Dear God, help me through this, I prayed. My left arm was beginning to tingle as the nurse ushered me into the examining room. My eyes opened wide in fear when I saw the doctor already seated and waiting for me. He had what looked like x-ray films in his hand.

"I'm sorry, Mrs. Carducci … " he began.

I didn't want to believe what I was hearing. My knees felt weak and I had to sit down.

"Are you all right?" he asked, noticing my distress.

"I'm fine." My mouth had gone dry and my voice sounded tinny. "What did you find?"

"I'm sorry you had to wait so long to hear this, but I wanted to be absolutely sure before I shared the good news."

"Good news? You have good news?" I asked. Was he really saying that?

"Yes. I'm happy to report that there is no sign you had, or ever will have, a stroke. Nor have you had any seizures. Here, take a look at this."

He placed two of the films side by side on the light board and, using his pen, traced the arteries shown on them. "See this clear pathway here? That's what I call beautiful. There's no plaque buildup to break loose and cause any problems. I wish all my patients had blood vessels that look like that. Your heart checks out fine as well. All your tests are normal. I'm pleased to say you're in very good health."

So it's G.O.K. after all?" I couldn't hide my relief at hearing the good news, or my disappointment at not having an answer.

"No. It's not G.O.K. What you're having is a form of migraine."

"But I've had migraines in the past. They're excruciatingly painful. There's no pain with these spells. I used to have migraines, but they stopped after I was divorced. I haven't had one in years."

"When you divorced, you removed the trigger for your migraines, but you didn't remove the propensity. You end a bad marriage and stress levels drop. The migraines go away. Like most people these days, your stress levels have increased, and with that your migraines are back. I'm pleased to hear you aren't having pain. If you do have pain in the future, come back and see me and we can deal with it then."

"What do I do for now?"

"Try to reduce your stress, relax as often as possible, and continue to take good care of yourself. If you feel you need a mild tranquilizer, I can prescribe one."

I thought of all the tranquilizers and mood enhancers Rodger had taken for so many years. Some of them were considered the miracle drugs of their day, the side effects of long-term use not clearly understood until much later.

"I don't want to start on them if I can avoid it. If things get worse, I'll let you know."

"Okay, then, good luck to you both. I'm here if you need me, but I hope you don't," the doctor said with a smile.

Grateful for the good news, Mike and I walked to the car holding hands, thankful to have each other.

"Life is good," Mike said, turning to give me a kiss before starting the car.

"Yes, it is," I agreed, kissing him right back. "Now all I have to do is figure out how to relax more and keep the migraines from escalating into the debilitating kind. I don't have time for them."

That evening I was taking a hot shower before bed, giving my hair a final rinse to remove all the rich lather, when I realized the water was pooling around my feet. Looking down, I discovered several strands of my hair blocking the drain. I refused to accept that this was another symptom of stress and pretended the new shampoo I was using was still too harsh or the water was too hot. Adjusting the mix to cool, I rinsed the rest of the soap out as gently as possible. I made a mental note to get a bottle of baby shampoo the next time I went to the store. Maybe that would help.

Chapter 23

Despite all that I did, even with Jackson's help, Rodger's health continued to decline. His C.O.P.D. was the cause of most of his problems. Chronic bronchitis would evolve into pneumonia very fast and he'd end up back in the hospital, always in isolation because of the MRSA. At least I knew he wouldn't be in danger of wandering off. MRSA patients have to stay in their rooms. In between hospital stays there were appointments with his psychiatrist, cardiologist, neurologist, urologist, podiatrist, dentist, and eye doctor. A symptom or ailment needing treatment occurred on an almost-weekly basis, and every holiday he'd crash and end up in the hospital. His behavior became more and more erratic.

One day I was doing some housework when I noticed the odor of something burning coming from Rodger's room. Terrified, I raced down the hall to save him, all the while wondering what could have caused a fire.

"What's up?" he asked, looking up from the TV.

Relief flooded through me when I realized there was no fire. Not yet anyway.

"What are you doing?" I demanded, anger replacing my fear.

I grabbed the smoking paper towel he'd draped over the bare bulb of the lamp on his side table. The shade was sitting on the floor at his feet.

"I use it to wipe my eyes. I have to dry the paper somehow."

"Are you kidding me?" I tried not to shout.

Think of him as a child. Calmly explain what he should do when his paper towel gets wet.

I sat down beside him and spoke softly. "It's dangerous to put paper towels on the light bulb. The paper will burn and you could get hurt. When the paper towel gets wet, throw it away and use another one."

"Nothing happened. You worry too much. I don't want to waste the paper towels."

"It's okay. We have plenty of paper towels. Use as many as you need. Promise me, no more paper towels on the light bulb. We don't want anyone to get hurt. You could set the house on fire."

"Yeah, yeah, no more paper towels on the light bulb. I get it."

Unfortunately, that wasn't the end of it. I entered his room several times to find the same thing happening. Eventually I took his paper towels and tissues away and insisted he use a handkerchief to wipe his eyes. He had a stack of them in a dresser drawer; he might as well use them. I warned him that they, while stronger than paper, could still burn and he wasn't to put them on the light bulb. When he still didn't stop, and I found a scorched handkerchief in his laundry basket one morning, I removed the lamp from his room and replaced it with a freestanding one that was too tall for him to reach the bulb. He didn't say anything when I took the lamp away, but his glower of resentment revealed how he felt.

One Saturday afternoon I heard him going into the bathroom every few minutes. Each time he'd go to the sink and run the water for a few minutes and go back to his room. When I went up to find out what was going on, I found him on the couch with a bloody handkerchief hanging out of his mouth.

"What happened?"

He shook his head and pointed at the handkerchief to indicate he couldn't talk.

"Please, open your mouth and let me see where the blood is coming from."

After several shakes of his head and my continued insistence, he finally gave in and removed the cloth, revealing a long gash in his tongue.

"How did this happen?" I asked. His only response was a shrug.

A few minutes later, Rodger, Mike, and I were on our way to the local urgent care office. There the doctor discovered that his partial plate had broken and a sharp wire had cut his tongue. He put in a few stitches and sent us home, instructing Rodger to keep the denture out of his moth until it could be repaired or replaced.

On Monday I called and made an appointment for him to see his dentist. Despite reporting the cut and his inability to use the partial plate until it was repaired, we had to wait a week to see a dentist. Until then I kept the plate with me so I wouldn't forget it. We were in the car on the way to his appointment when Rodger asked if I remembered to bring it.

"Yes, it's in my purse."

Five minutes later he asked the same question and I reminded him I had it. A short time later he asked again so I reached into my purse and pulled out of the storage case and showed it to him.

"See, it's right here. There's no need to worry."

"I don't worry about anything," he answered. "Give it to me," he said, holding out his hand.

"It's okay in my purse."

"It's mine. Give it to me," he insisted.

Exasperated at this insistence, and hoping to avoid upsetting him even more, I handed it over.

"You can hold it but don't put it on your mouth. It's broken and it will cut you again."

"How do you know?"

"It cut you once already, remember?"

"I remember. Maybe today it won't cut me. I have to try." He opened the case.

"Close the case and hold it until the dentist looks at it. If he can fix it, you can put it on your mouth later."

I wondered why he was so insistent on putting it in. He often took it out overnight and would have to insert it at mealtime.

Reluctantly he closed the case again. A few seconds later, he popped it open and tried to put the darned thing in his mouth again.

"Rodger, stop. Don't do that. It will cut your tongue."

"You think you know everything. It won't cut me this time."

Not willing to take that chance, I reached over and took it. I continued to hold onto it until we entered the treatment room where I handed it over to the dental assistant.

"She stole my teeth." Rodger said to the woman. "She took them so I can't eat. She wants me to starve to death. She's crazy."

The only response from the technician was a raised eyebrow and a questioning look directed at me.

No wonder my hair is falling out and I'm having weird migraines, I thought. Ignoring his accusation, I explained about the cut to his tongue and why I was keeping his teeth from him.

Rodger repeated his accusation when the dentist entered the room. He either didn't hear him or pretended not to. After checking Rodger's teeth and assessing the damage to the device, he told Rodger that he couldn't repair it. His gums had receded so it didn't fit anymore. Any repair he did now would only be temporary as it would break again.

"You don't give me my teeth?"

"Not yet. We'll take impressions today, and in a few weeks you'll come back and get the new one. It will fit better and feel a lot better too. Okay?"

"Do what you want. I have no choice. She's in charge."

Taking that as agreement, the dentist told me I'd receive a call when it was time to bring him to be fitted, and he left the room.

Again, Rodger was quiet all the way home, and he didn't speak to me when I took him his afternoon medication. All afternoon I listened to him pacing. He didn't turn on the TV or take his usual midday nap.

Oh boy, I thought. He's really upset about this. We're in for it now.

When Mike came in the door, he seemed to know immediately something was wrong. "What is it this time?" he said, exasperation clear in his tone.

I lifted my hand in warning. "Stop right there," I said, and walked away.

I wasn't in the mood to be questioned or criticized, and if that was going to be his attitude, I wanted no part of him or his father.

Mike's response whenever he knew I was this upset was to keep quiet and run away. He'd give me some time to cool down before hearing me out. He'd made it halfway up the stairs to change when Rodger called out to him.

"I need my teeth. She won't give my teeth!"

"Your plate is broken. It cut you. Didn't you go to the dentist today?" Mike asked.

"I went. The dentist won't give me my teeth either. He does what she says."

"He's probably going to fix them for you. You just have to wait a few days."

"I can't wait. I have to eat sometime. If I don't get a sandwich soon, I'm going to be a goner. You don't listen. Nobody listens. She doesn't feed me all day."

"What do you mean, she doesn't feed you? She makes food for you every day. Did you have breakfast today?"

"No breakfast. No lunch. She never gives me food."

I had heard enough. "This is the same shit he told the dentist today. I can't believe this. He had scrambled eggs and toast for breakfast. For lunch he ate mashed potatoes, carrots, and chicken. And even though he said he didn't want it, I left him a pudding cup for a snack later. I pointed to the empty container and the plastic spoon on the side table."

"Did you eat that pudding?" Mike asked.

"No."

"Who did?"

"Maybe she did. She tries to fool you. You always take her side. She controls you and she tries to control me."

I tried to hold back my anger and frustration, but it wasn't to be this time.

"Why the hell would I spend part of each day cooking things you like? Things that are good for you. Do I do that just so I can let you starve? You can't have your effing teeth because they'll cut your mouth, and then you really won't be able to eat. It's not going to kill you to go a few days without them. Goddammit, Rodger. You are a selfish, ungrateful man who lies about me all the time. I try so hard to make you happy and keep you alive, and you fight me as if I'm your enemy. I think you love the drama. You stir things up on purpose just for the fun of it."

"See, she's crazy. Listen to her holler at me."

"No wonder she hollers at you," Mike shouted. "You know she loves you. You know we're both doing everything we can for you. Why do you do this to us?"

"I don't do anything to you. You think I do this on purpose? She has you fooled. That's what."

Suddenly all the anger and resentment drained out of me to be replaced by profound sadness. I had failed him again and allowed my weakness to influence Mike's feelings as well. What were we doing arguing with him? He believed what he was saying. If he denied having his breakfast and lunch with such vehemence, it must mean he had forgotten he ate them. Add in keeping his teeth away from him, and I could understand his panic.

"This is getting us nowhere," I told Mike. "You go get changed and I'll fix a plate for him. Maybe then he'll settle down. It won't hurt him to have another meal. And it will give me time to think about what to do to keep this from happening again."

"I'm sorry I snapped at you earlier," Mike said after an almost-silent meal. Rodger was snoring loudly in his room after eating only a few bites of his second dinner.

"Don't waste it," Rodger said when I went up to take the dishes away. "I'll eat it tomorrow."

"Okay. Let me know if you want a snack later. If not, I'll see you in the morning." All the anger and suspicion seemed to have left him, and I vowed to find a way to keep it that way.

"I hate what's happening to us. We don't treat each other like that," I said in response to Mike's apology.

He took my hand and gave it an affectionate squeeze. "I know it's hard for you but I need a few minutes to decompress when I get home. I hate it when you jump at me the minute I walk in. I'm happy to listen once I get changed and shake off the workday. Until then, I'm just not ready to hear about the disaster of the day."

I could have jumped on him for the insensitive way he expressed his need for time alone when he got home, but I didn't. There had been enough drama already, and I knew what he meant and I didn't blame him.

"Always remember we're in this together," he added.

"Yes we are," I said, but we both knew I was more in it than he was. I was the target of his father's suspicion, and I was the one who had to deal with it.

The next morning, when I served Rodger his breakfast, I handed him a small notebook and asked him write down what he had to eat and sign and date the entry.

"What's this for?" he asked.

"It's so you don't forget that you ate."

"I don't forget anything. I know when I eat."

"That's good," I answered cheerfully. "I'm glad to hear it. But we'll keep this log in case your doctor asks about your diet. We can show it to him so he knows you eat well."

"What I eat is none of his business. The food is good here. Everything is nice."

Yesterday I was starving him and controlling Mike. Today everything is nice. I'd take it and thank God he was having a good day.

After a relatively peaceful day and a quiet evening, I lay awake long after both men were asleep. I prayed for guidance and assistance. I knew that as hard as this was, it wouldn't last forever. If only I could figure out how to make him happy. I wanted his last days to be good ones. He'd endured enough hardship and loss in his life. I wondered why I always make so many mistakes in my relationships with the people I care about. For some reason I always fall short. I had let years go by with little or no contact with my mother. Thank God I resolved those issues in time. My father was somewhere out in the world with his new family, and I failed at my first marriage, causing deep pain for my children and me.

I was terrified I'd mess this up and not only lose Rodger, but Mike as well. How long would he continue to believe in me when each day brought another crisis? I didn't know what I was doing. I was making it up as I went along. There were many moments when I wanted to give up and tell Mike we had to admit his father to long-term care, just to save myself the worry and stress of it all, but I couldn't. Not when doing so would be a death sentence for Rodger. I wouldn't be able to live with myself if my weakness resulted in the death of someone so fragile.

Dear Lord, protect him from my mistakes. Hold us in your love and light and show me the way.

Chapter 24

I bolted awake. Something was very wrong. Was I dreaming? A powerful feeling of dread washed over me. My heart was pounding so hard I could see my nightgown moving with every beat. It felt as if an elephant were sitting on my chest. Not a nightmare. A heart attack!

"Mike, wake up. Wake up. I need your help!" I shook him as hard as I could, fear and confusion forcing adrenaline through my veins. My heart rate was increasing with every thought.

"What's happening? Is it Rodger?" Mike rose from the bed, stumbling as he tried to come awake and turn on the light.

"No, it's not Rodger. It's me. There's something wrong with my heart. Call 911."

As my heart continued to beat faster than I thought possible, I silently prayed that God would spare me.

I can't die like this. I can't do this to Mike or my children. Help me hang on until help can arrive. I want to live. Help me. Please help me.

I couldn't believe what I was seeing when I looked up and discovered Mike walking in circles at the foot of the bed, running his hands through his hair.

"Mike, call 911! I'm in trouble." I tried to shout but my voice came out barely above a whisper.

"I can't remember the number," was his plaintive reply.

"Pick up the phone and punch in the numbers 9-1-1. Do it now," I ordered him before lying down on the bed, hoping the change in position would ease the pressure in my chest.

How can he just stand there when I need him? I had never felt so alone. I was going to die while he stood helplessly by and watched.

Fortunately the sound of my voice snapped Mike out of his trance, and he was able to make the call. Several minutes later the ambulance arrived and the emergency team raced up the stairs and into my room. Within seconds I was given oxygen and hooked up to a portable EKG machine.

After checking and rechecking the readings, and listening to my heart and lungs, the paramedic reassured me I wasn't having a heart attack.

"You're going to be okay. If you were in danger, you'd see a lot more urgency in us. If we don't worry, you don't have to worry. Got it?"

"I get it." The oxygen had helped me breathe normally again, and the pressure in my chest was gone.

"This looks like a reaction to stress. What do you have in the house to help you calm down?" he asked.

"How about some vodka?" I joked.

"If that's what will do it, okay. And give some to your husband. He looks worse than you do."

"I think I feel worse than she does," Mike agreed. "I'm still shaking from the scare."

"Do you want to go to the hospital?" the paramedic asked me. "I don't think it's necessary, but if you feel the need to see a doctor, we'll be happy to take you."

"No. As long as I'm in no danger, I want to stay here."

"All right then. We'll pack up and get out of here and let you get some rest. You should follow up with your doctor tomorrow. And do what you can to reduce your stress level. It's not good for you or that man over there," he said, pointing to Mike. "If you need us again anytime, even if it's again tonight, you call us right away. Promise?"

"I promise."

After the ambulance pulled away, I looked at Mike, who appeared to have aged ten years in the last hour.

"I'm sorry I scared you, but I was pretty scared myself. I thought I was dying."

"I'm sorry you had to go through that," he answered. "Come here, let me hold you. I need to feel you in my arms. Please don't do that again. I couldn't bear to lose you."

"I don't plan on it. That was the scariest thing I ever felt. But, just in case, you should probably write 911 on your hand so you don't forget the number if you ever need it again."

I laughed with him at my little joke, but deep inside I wondered if I'd ever feel safe again, knowing that I can't count on him to rescue me when I need it.

The next morning I asked Rodger if he had a good night's sleep.

"I never closed an eye all night," he said.

"Really? So you heard the ambulance crew here last night?"

I knew he hadn't, as the paramedic had commented on the loud snoring coming from his room as they prepared to leave.

"An ambulance was here last night? They came for me?" he asked.

"No, for me," I said.

"What happened to you?"

"I was feeling sick, but I'm okay now." I didn't want to upset him with the details.

"Thank God you're okay," he said.

I was touched by his comment—until he completed his thought.

"If you go down, I go down, so I hope you stay healthy."

"So much for sentiment," I said, giving him a pat on the shoulder. "Let's hope we both stay healthy and then nobody has to worry."

"It's no use worrying. You're going to die one of these days. There's no escape. That's why I don't worry about nothing," he said. "So where's my breakfast. I have to eat sometime."

As far as Rodger was concerned, that was the end of it. For me, it was the beginning of another phase as a caregiver. As I fought to keep my father-in-law alive, my own health was suffering. Always without warning, the panic attacks continued. But now that I knew what they were, I fought through the panic. When I felt one coming on, I'd go to my room, sit on my bed, and take slow, deep breaths until the feeling passed. My doctor offered tranquilizers again, and again I refused. I would not give in to weakness and end up addicted to pills. I'd put on my big girl panties and deal with it.

Thanksgiving would arrive soon, and I was looking forward to it. The house would be full of company. Two of our children were coming with their families, and my cousin and her husband were making a rare trip to the area and would be staying with us for a few days. Every year I looked forward to cooking the holiday meal. Even though it would mean more work, I knew the break in routine, and time spent with family, laughing and telling stories, would be good for me.

When the day finally arrived, I was thrilled that things were going so well. My cousin and her husband are fun to have around. Mike always said he loved listening to me laugh, and when he saw me relaxing and giggling at the jokes they told, he joined in with gusto. Even Rodger seemed to be having a good time when he ventured out of his room for breakfast and lunch. Despite the holiday, he'd keep to his routine, but I hoped he'd join us at the table for dessert later.

My homemade apple and pumpkin pies were sitting out on the counter. The potatoes were peeled and ready to be cooked when the time came. The aroma of roasting turkey and stuffing wafted through the house. When the wind picked up outside, Mike lit a fire in the fireplace, and everyone gathered in the family room to enjoy a cocktail or two before dinner. We could hear the wind whistling between the houses and watched the trees outside the window bow almost in half.

Mike offered a toast. "To Thanksgiving and to being safe and warm with our family on this holiday."

"Here, here," everyone agreed.

And then the power went out.

"Don't worry," he told everyone. "This happens every now and then. It will probably come back on soon."

No one seemed bothered by the outage, especially after I placed candles in every room and made sure Rodger had his flashlight. The family room looked lovely, and no one objected to the idea of dining by candlelight. The only problem would be how to finish cooking the turkey when the oven was out.

"Come on, power company," I urged. "I have a house full of hungry people here."

When two hours passed and it was clear the wind wasn't about to die down and the power could be out for a long time, we decided to put the turkey on the grill to finish cooking it.

"We have salad, deviled eggs, and cranberry sauce to go with it for now. We can cook the potatoes and other side dishes tomorrow with the leftover turkey. And there's pie for dessert," I said, trying to put the best spin on the situation.

Everyone agreed it would be fine. But poor Mike was the one who had to brave the wind on the deck to put the turkey on. He removed the stuffing and set it aside to bake later, and cut the turkey in half so it would cook faster.

He managed to get it done.

As we sat down to eat, everyone agreed he was the hero of the day. Rodger decided not to join us for dessert after all. He said he was full and I didn't push it. He was never comfortable around a lot of people, and I'd take him a small piece of each pie later.

I had excused myself to freshen up after dinner when I heard Mike calling me.

"Did you need something?" I asked, coming into the room.

"My dad's looking for you. He said his chest hurts. It's probably heartburn, but I told him you'd be up to check on him."

I went up immediately, stopping to gather up my stethoscope, blood pressure monitor, and thermometer on the way. I knew Jackson would be home celebrating Thanksgiving with his family, so there was no point in hooking up the telehealth monitor.

"Mike said your chest hurts. Is that right?" I said upon entering Rodger's room.

"Yes, it hurts. I feel heavy."

"How long have you had this pain?" I asked.

"Since I ate supper."

I looked at my watch. It was 8:30 p.m. He'd eaten promptly at 4:00, as usual.

"You've been in pain for four and half hours? Why didn't you tell me?"

"I didn't want to bother you. You have company."

"It's not a bother to me when you need help. That's what I'm here for. I'm glad you called for me now."

I took his wrist in my hand and felt for a pulse. I couldn't seem to place my fingers in the right spot to get a reading. This had never happened before, but rather than worry about it, I put the stethoscope over his heart to have a listen. I couldn't hear anything. His heart had to be beating because he was sitting up, talking to me. I tried again and again. Still no sound. *There must be something wrong with the stethoscope,* I thought. Fortunately I had another one. After retrieving it and trying again with the same result, I got scared. Not wanting to let on to him how serious I thought this was, I told him to sit tight and I'd be right back. Then I went downstairs and called 911.

"911 what's your emergency?"

"I have a 75-year-old male with chest pain, and I can't get a reading of his pulse. And I can't hear his heartbeat, even with my stethoscope. I know he has one because he's sitting up and talking. Please send an ambulance."

I answered all the operator's questions, provided the address, and went back upstairs to sit with Rodger until the paramedics arrived. The mood in the house was no longer festive. Everyone gathered in the family room, silently hoping that Rodger would be okay.

"He's in complete blockage," the paramedic stated to the EMTs with him. "I'm going to administer a clot buster and within two minutes he's going to pink up nicely. In the meantime get ready to transport him. He's not to lift a finger to help. Move him onto the stretcher and keep him warm. Let's go."

As the EMTs prepared to take Rodger to the hospital, the paramedic turned to me and said, "His heart was hardly beating at all. If he had waited even a few more minutes before letting you know he needed help, he'd be gone now."

"I guess that's why I couldn't feel a pulse or hear his heartbeat."

"That's right," he said. "We're taking him to the nearest hospital. You can follow us if you like. And bring along a list of his medications. The ER doctor will need to see it."

As Mike drove us to the hospital, I wished I had been allowed to go with Rodger in the ambulance. From my own recent scare, I knew he must be terrified. I didn't want him to be alone with his fear. I didn't want him to die. Yes he was difficult and I often cracked under the strain, but I loved him. I knew the gentle soul that lived within him. I treasured the quiet dignity that emerged in the rare moments of clarity I had the privilege to witness. If this was to be the end, I wanted to be with him. He had become as precious to me as my own missing father.

Soon after arriving at the hospital, Mike and I were informed that arrangements were being made to transport Rodger to a larger hospital, one with an excellent cardiac care unit, where a surgeon was standing by to operate immediately.

"Under normal conditions, we'd call for a life flight helicopter to take him, but with the wind whipping around out there, it's impossible," the doctor said.

Hours later we sat in silence in the waiting room waiting for word on his condition. Would we always remember this holiday as the day we lost him, or would we have a real reason for giving thanks?

At first the news was good. He came through the surgery well. A stent was inserted and his heart was beating fine.

"He's a lucky man. If he had to have a heart attack, this was the kind to have. There isn't a lot of damage to the muscle, and he probably won't need a pacemaker. We'll keep an eye on him for a few days and then send him home."

After getting home and reporting the good news to everyone, Mike and I went to bed, thanking God for another miracle.

Unfortunately the doctor's hopeful prognosis didn't hold up. The heart attack did more damage than originally thought. A few days later he underwent surgery to implant a pacemaker. The doctor was surprised again when, instead of pacing occasionally as he had thought, the pacemaker had to work constantly to keep him alive.

The surgeries and medications took a huge toll on Rodger, both physically and mentally. He was often confused, thinking he was back in Italy resisting the Gestapo. At other times it was clear he was hearing voices. His swallowing problem returned and was more severe than ever. I stayed at his bedside from early morning until evening. I knew that even in the best of hospitals, patients need an advocate to communicate with doctors and nurses.

His bed was placed directly across from the nurses' station so he could be monitored through the night. Still he managed to remove his IV, catheter, and heart monitor, and strip off his clothes when no one was looking. He'd wander the halls naked, speaking in Italian. Only when I arrived would he settle down and go to sleep. When both his younger son and his very busy brother came to visit, he became convinced he was going to die. Why else would they bother to come? After everyone else left and he and I were alone, he'd cry silently and hold my hand. In those moments we didn't have to speak. I understood his fear and confusion, as well as his need for simple human touch. For most of his life his fractured mind had left him unable to tolerate closeness, while his body and soul cried out for it. With that simple gesture he communicated that he trusted me to take care of him. I'd keep that trust, no matter how difficult it became.

Chapter 25

"I want a sandwich," Rodger demanded when I took him his lunch.

In the month since coming home from the hospital, he had gained some weight, and the home nurse was no longer coming every day to check on him. The better he felt, the more he complained about the pureed food he was forced to eat, and the walker he had to use.

"I know you do," I replied, placing the bowl of homemade black bean soup on the tray table in front of him. "I wish you could have one, but you wouldn't be able to swallow it. You'll choke and food will go into your lungs and make you sick."

"Don't be stupid! Food can't go into lungs. Give me some real food."

"Try this soup. I think you'll like it. I made it this morning."

I handed him a child-size spoon and watched as he put it into his mouth. Before he could take a second bite, I placed my fingers on his wrist, holding the spoon down, and told him to swallow three times and count to ten before taking another bite.

Rodger sighed in frustration. "You treat me like a baby. I know how to eat."

"I wish we didn't have to do this, but we must. It's doctor's orders," I said, hoping to deflect some of the anger he was feeling.

The two things Rodger enjoyed most were eating and walking, and now both had been taken away from him. Parkinson's disease and residual damage from the heart attack left him at high risk of falling, making a walker necessary. He was never to use the stairs unless Mike or I were there to help him. I agreed to take his meals and medications up to him, so there was no need for him to leave the second floor. He hated the restriction and he hated the walker, and I didn't blame him. Still, I had to follow the doctor's advice and keep him safe.

The throat specialist confirmed that his swallowing problem had worsened, and he'd never be able to eat solid food again. Everything he ate had to be pureed, and liquids had to be thickened to the consistency of honey. It was critical that he take very small bites and chew thoroughly. He'd always be at risk of aspiration. Even if he followed instructions to the letter, he could choke on his own saliva.

None of it made sense to Rodger. Food doesn't go to your lungs, it goes to your stomach. That meant someone was trying to keep him from eating, and I was in on it. He insisted he didn't need a walker. When I wasn't looking, he'd sneak out of his room and walk down the hall without it. He didn't fall. He didn't die. Something was very wrong in this house, and I wasn't to be trusted.

"I'm going to tell the doctor the next time we go," he told me almost daily.

"That's fine. Tell the doctor anything you want. If something worries you, you should tell him," I always responded. "Do you want to write it down so you don't forget?"

"I don't forget nothing. I don't have to write it down. I'm going to tell the doctor next time. You wait and see."

And so it goes, I thought as I watched and counted as he ate his soup. I worked hard to make his meals as nutritious as possible, using fresh ingredients and lots of herbs and spices. My concoctions often came out looking like gruel, but I always tested them to make sure they tasted good. Jackson and Rodger's doctors were surprised by my creativity. I could puree almost anything, pickles being one exception. From roast beef with roasted vegetables to hot dogs and potato salad, I found a way to make it work. For dessert, I sometimes pureed a cupcake, and for lunch one afternoon I pureed a tuna salad and tomato sandwich. I severely overcooked macaroni and added homemade sauce so he could even have the pasta he loved. But I couldn't give him what he really craved: a nice thick sandwich and a big, juicy orange. The pita bread he loved was no longer allowed, and he'd never eat a bowl of cereal again. His long walks outside were a thing of the past. No wonder he was angry and suspicious. I was treating him like a child. The sad part was, I had no choice and it would never get better.

"Let me see your hand," I said the next morning when Rodger reached for the spoon to eat his breakfast.

"What's the matter?" he asked.

"It's swollen. Does it hurt?"

"No."

"Did you bump it?"

"No. You worry too much. Sometimes your hand swells, that's all."

I knew better than to argue. I let it go while he ate his breakfast. Soon after I checked his vital signs and sent them to the hospital for Jackson to read. Everything looked pretty good, but I decided to give him a call anyway and tell him about the swelling. Jackson wasn't concerned when I told him of the puffiness in Rodger's fingers and hand. He said to keep an eye on it and keep him posted if it seemed to be worsening. When I went up to check on him an hour later, the hand looked slightly larger than before but I wasn't sure. I got a tape measure and measured both wrists. The left one was a quarter of an inch larger than the right. *No big deal,* I thought and went on about my morning routine. An hour later when I checked him again, the difference had increased to a full inch and the swelling was moving up his arm. I called Jackson again, but he was away from his desk and I got the answering machine. I waited thirty minutes and checked Rodger's arm again. This time I didn't need a measuring tape to tell me the swelling had increased and was moving up his arm. I called Jackson and left a message, telling him I was taking Rodger to the emergency room and we should be there within the hour.

By the time we arrived at the hospital, his entire arm, from fingers to shoulder, was swollen. It looked twice the size of the other one. He was admitted to the hospital immediately with a suspected blood clot. A Doppler ultrasound confirmed it. He would be in the hospital for several days on high doses of blood thinners to dissolve the clots, and he'd remain on blood thinners after his release. That would mean weekly trips to the hospital to have his blood checked to determine how fast his blood was clotting and whether or not his medication had to be adjusted. We were told when the pacemaker was inserted that a possible side effect could be increased chance of blood clotting. I should have expected this. With Rodger, if anything could go wrong, it would. I couldn't help but wonder how much more his body could take.

I sat with him every day as his blood was monitored and the clots began to break up. The swelling in his arm was almost gone and plans were being made to send him home. I was pleased to note he seemed happy with that idea. I was packing a bag with the clothes he'd wear home when the phone rang.

It was Jackson and he had bad news. "Bobbi, I'm sorry to tell you this, but Rodger won't be going home for a while. He's pretty sick."

"What happened? He was fine when I left last night."

"He developed a fever and started coughing during the night. He has pneumonia. He was moved to the fourth floor where he's being treated for it. We hope he responds to the medication quickly, but there's no way he can go home today."

"Thanks for letting me know. I'll be in to see him in a little while."

"Hang in there and call me if you need anything," Jackson said before hanging up.

I sat on Rodger's bed, looking at the overnight bag holding his clothes. *Why, Lord?* I asked. *Why does he have to go through so much? He was happy to be coming home, and I was looking forward to being home and not having to drive for forty minutes twice a day to watch over him. God, I'm so tired I just want to lie down on this bed and sleep for a week.*

"Are you ready?" Mike called upstairs to me. It was his day off and we had planned to pick him up together.

"I'm ready but he's not."

Minutes later, after explaining this latest setback, we were on our way to the hospital.

After donning gown and gloves to enter his isolation room, I took a moment to take a deep breath and put a smile on my face. I didn't want him to see my concern. He was far too fragile to take even a mild pneumonia lightly.

My expression turned to one of shock and anger when I saw him. He greeted us with a rare smile, seemingly unaware of how terrible he looked. His face and neck were covered with little cuts, and blood was seeping from most of them. There was even a cut on the tip of his nose.

"What happened to you?" I demanded. I was shaking with anger.

"Nothing happened to me. I want to go home. Did you come to take me home?"

"You have to stay a few more days. You have a fever," Mike explained.

"Look at this," I said, my fury mounting by the second.

"Why is she so mad?" Rodger asked Mike.

"This is why." I pointed to the razor sitting on the tray alongside leftovers from his breakfast. "Look, there's blood on the blades. And look at what they gave him for breakfast. Orange juice, toast, scrambled eggs, and fried potatoes." After spotting a large Styrofoam cup of ice water with a straw sticking out of it, I turned and stormed out of the room, gown and gloves still on.

"I need to speak to the nurse in charge right now," I informed the only person at he desk who bothered to acknowledge my presence.

"You can't be walking around here in that gown. Dispose of it properly in the waste container before leaving the patient's room. It's important that everyone follow the rules. I believe you've been here often enough to know that."

"I know the importance of following the rules. I also know the importance of reading a patient's chart before giving him dangerous items or food that he can't swallow. Now find the person in charge of this floor and the patient advocate and tell them I demand to speak with them. I'll be waiting in Mr. Carducci's room."

"Don't listen to her," Rodger said to the head nurse as soon as she entered his room. "She worries too much. Go take care of the sick people"

"What seems to be the problem here?" she asked me.

"Let's start with the cuts on his face and neck, shall we?" I began. "Look at him. He's a mess. Why was a patient with Parkinson's disease, who is also on blood thinners, given a razor?"

"I can see why you're upset by this but, trust me, the cuts are superficial and he's in no danger."

"Excuse me? You think this is okay? The fact that blood is oozing from those cuts is of no concern? Did you ever nick yourself shaving your legs? It hurts and he has dozens of them. I can't believe you aren't as appalled by this as we are."

"Believe me, I am concerned. I will find out what happened and see to it he isn't given a razor again, but you have to calm down."

"I'll calm down when I'm assured he's not in danger of hurting himself. The razor is the most visible problem but not the only one. He has severe dysphagia. He can't swallow properly. All his food must be pureed. He is never to use a straw. His meals are to be supervised to make sure he doesn't choke and aspirate. Look at the tray they gave him this morning. Toast, of all things, and chunks of potato. He can't have orange juice or any other liquid unless it's been thickened. And there on his bedside table is a large cup of water. Listen to him speak. There is clearly a liquid buildup in his throat. It sounds like he's talking under water. All he has to do is cough and it will go right into his lungs. Didn't anyone read his chart? And please tell me you're crushing his medications and mixing them with applesauce, as directed. If not, he could end up having a mental break if he's here for very long."

To her credit the nurse listened quietly until I ran out of steam.

"I understand your distress, and I am very concerned by what you're telling me. I'm going to review his chart, and when I've finished I'd like the two of you to come to my office where we can talk about this and take steps to see that the situation is corrected. Everyone here wants what's best for your father."

I didn't bother telling her that if she had read the chart she'd know he's not my father.

The woman returned a few minutes later and taped large, handprinted signs above Rodger's bed. NO RAZORS, PUREED FOOD AND THICKENED LIQUIDS ONLY, NO STRAWS, MEDS CRUSHED IN APPLESAUCE.

When the last one was in place, she turned and left again, saying, "I'll have a nurse let you know when I'm ready to meet with you.

"Mr. and Mrs. Carducci, my main purpose here is to see to it that your father gets the best care we can offer. It's him I'm concerned about. So I'm not worried about your distress or hurting your feelings when I say you overreacted when addressing my staff. You were rude and demanding and I won't have that.

"He was admitted to this ward last night. Neither one of you was here to speak with the staff about his special needs or your concerns. It's important for family members to stick around until the patient is settled in and not drop them off like so much baggage. We took care of him overnight, and this morning we gave him his breakfast and provided him with items for his personal hygiene. You can't blame us if he didn't follow his diet and took it upon himself to shave."

"Oh boy, you're in for it now," Mike said to the nurse. "From the look in my wife's eye, I know you just added fuel to her anger."

"Where is the patient advocate?" I asked. "I want her here as well."

"She's not in today. But I will make her aware of the situation as soon as I can."

"When you do," I spoke very slowly and clearly, "Make sure you inform her that we did not drop him off like baggage. You inform her he was transferred to your ward from the ICU where he was being treated for blood clots in his arm that developed after insertion of a pacemaker. You inform her that he suffered a heart attack on Thanksgiving Day. You see to it that she understands that he suffers from Parkinson's disease, schizophrenia, and age-related dementia, and that the pneumonia he has now was most likely caused by aspiration due to his dysphagia—and your staff may have made it worse today.

"You inform her that he has been a VA hospital patient since 1947 and a patient here for six years, and that his case is one of the most complicated you will ever come across. His combination of illnesses demand constant attention, and his chart should come up with a red flag on every page, warning hospital personnel of the danger he can be to himself if he wanders off, and the risks of leaving him unattended at meals. You make sure everyone knows he is not to be given razors or straws or laxatives.

"Will you do that when you speak to her? Will you do what I have done every day for six years and then sit in that chair and lecture me on how I wasn't present when he arrived on your ward last night? How dare you suggest that we are less than responsible when you are speaking from inexcusable ignorance of the patient you say is your main priority?"

I sat back in my chair, exhausted and in tears, wondering if I had just made things worse. I needed these people. There were times when I had to leave him in their care. I couldn't afford to alienate them.

The nurse looked at me in stunned silence. Nobody moved for several seconds, and then Mike did what only he would do in a situation like that. He rose to his feet and began clapping.

"Bravo, my darling, well done!"

At first I couldn't believe my ears, and then I discovered I was laughing through my tears. I fell in love with him all over again in that moment. What woman wouldn't adore a man who supported her fully, even when she made an ass of herself.

"Well," the nurse finally spoke, "I can see your father has a fierce advocate in you, and I will see to it that everyone treating him is aware of your concerns. I assure you we want him to get the best possible care."

"I've said this before and I'm saying it again, I know that no one here is deliberately careless. I know that you have many patients to care for and you are often shorthanded. I get it. But you have all his records at your fingertips in that computerized system of yours, and it does him no good if no one reads it. Just make sure they read it, so I can leave his bedside long enough to get some sleep while he's here."

"I will," she promised, and the so-called meeting was over.

I slept fitfully that night, twice awakening to breathe through threatening panic attacks. While waiting for sleep to take me between attacks, I prayed the same prayer I'd been repeating for weeks.

Dear Lord, I need help. Please send help any way you see fit. The words had almost become a mantra I repeated them so often. Day after day, week after week, I looked to God for help to no avail. Still I kept it up. *Please , God, I need help. Please send help.*

When I awoke, it was to discover an ice storm had swept through during the night. Schools and businesses were closed, and everyone was warned to stay off the roads. There was no way I could make the drive over mountain roads to the hospital. I called Jackson and asked him to check in on Rodger throughout the day. He assured me he would and told me to take advantage of the storm to get some much-needed rest.

"You know, Bobbi, when my time comes and I need someone to take care of me, I'm going to call you. I wish all my patients had someone to fight for them the way you fight for Rodger."

I chuckled. "So you heard about my tirade, did you?"

"I did, and I heard what Mike did as well. I agree with him. Bravo, girl! Now don't worry about Rodger. I'll visit with him right after I get off the phone and give him your love."

"Thank you, and tell him I'll give him a call later."

The temperature rose through the day, and by the next morning the sun was shining and the roads were clear. Jackson had called the evening before to reassure me and let me know that the pneumonia was responding to treatment. If he continued to improve, Rodger would be home by the weekend. Pleased to hear the good news, I also knew things would be chaotic for days as they always were when he came home after a stay in the hospital.

Are you listening, God? I need your help. Any way you see fit is fine with me.

I drove along the mountain pass, praying and hoping to find that everything the nurse had promised had come to pass. I was hoping for the best but preparing for the worst when the scenery began to change.

While the road was clear and the sun was shining brightly, every blade of grass, every twig on every branch of every tree I passed for miles, was encased in ice. I couldn't believe the beauty that was unfolding before me.

Tears filled my eyes and I felt an amazing sense of peace. *It's like driving through heaven.* Just as that thought came to mind, the song on the radio changed. The words filled me with awe, "There are angels among us."

I knew in that moment my prayers would be answered. Maybe not right away. Maybe not in the time I hoped for, but I knew I was not alone.

When I got to the hospital, I was told a social worker wanted to speak with me. Bracing for another lecture on how I was out of line for speaking my mind, I was shocked when the first thing he said was, "Mrs. Carducci, do you need help?"

"What did you say?" I asked, not sure I heard right.

"I asked if you need help. I understand that you've been caring for your father in your home for a long time and that his needs are extensive. Are you able to leave him to go to the store or go out to dinner with your husband? When was the last time you took an afternoon for yourself?"

"Um ..." I stuttered. "Wow. Yes, I need help. Who are you again?" I wanted to ask him to turn around so I could check for wings, but I was afraid to appear cheeky to God.

"Here's my card. My name is Rob Angelis, and I'm a social worker. I'd like to arrange some help for you. Mr. Carducci has a 100% disability rating, and I can offer you in-home assistance if you're willing to accept it."

"Oh, I'm willing to accept it." I said a silent prayer of thanks before continuing. "Please tell me more about the program and when we can start."

I was given the name of the person in charge of the program, and within hours a caseworker was assigned to us. He immediately authorized fourteen hours of home assistance by a local health provider. All I needed to do was talk to Mike and decide how we wanted to divide the time.

I'd use some hours during the week to go grocery shopping or get my hair done, anything I wanted to do. We'd take a few hours on the weekend to go out for dinner or a movie. We could even go to church together again. I was almost dancing with joy when I entered Rodger's room. My sense of relief intensified when I saw a nurse's aide monitoring him as he took a small spoonful of applesauce into his mouth."

"That's good, Mr. Carducci. Make sure you swallow three times to get all your medicine in you. Now let's count together," she said. "One, two, three."

Sometimes you have to turn up the volume if you want to get attention, even when you're talking to God.

Chapter 26

I was getting ready for bed after a long day of trying to keep track of Rodger. He'd been home and pneumonia-free for three months, and it was clear the latest illness had weakened him even more. Even using the walker to steady himself, it was hard for him to get up from a chair. At times his legs threatened to give out when he tried to walk; his right hand shook constantly. He'd falter and bump into walls when trying to go to the bathroom. It was a miracle he hadn't fallen. Several times I found him standing at the top of the stairs, rocking on unsteady legs. A fall would surely kill him, if not right away, then slowly and painfully from the consequences of a broken hip. One day, when the respite caregiver was with him, I went shopping and came back with a safety gate and baby monitor to allow me to keep an eye on him from anywhere in the house.

"What's that for?" he asked when I secured the gate.

"It's there to remind you not to go down the stairs alone."

"Take it away. I'll stay up here. Don't worry about me."

"It has to stay there. If you wake up in the night to go to the bathroom, you might get dizzy or get too close to the edge and fall down the steps."

My words didn't explain why I kept it up all the time, but I hoped the reason I gave him would satisfy him for a little while.

We were visiting the doctor for a checkup shortly after I set up the monitor, and Rodger said, "I can't get anything past this woman. She's on to me all the time."

It took him a couple of weeks to figure out that the little black device sitting on the shelf in his room was a camera.

When I told the doctor and Jackson how I managed to keep an eye on him, they were pleased and impressed by my ingenuity.

I was about to slip under the covers when I saw movement on the monitor. Rodger was headed toward the bathroom, his walker nowhere in sight.

"Don't forget your walker," I called out, heading for the door to intercept him.

I was halfway down the hall when the phone started ringing. Mike was out of town for work. We had spoken just a little while ago so I ignored it, letting the answering machine pick up. Although he'd walked only a few feet, by the time I reached him Rodger was shaking, whether from the Parkinson's disease or exertion, I didn't know. I steadied him and walked him to the bathroom and, when he had finished, back to his room.

After getting him settled, I sat and talked with him for a while. He was in rare form that evening. He talked for almost two hours about life in Italy. He told of taking a mule into town for supplies and how the animal balked at leaving the farm.

"I had to hit it with a switch to keep it moving to get there. Then the damn thing would run all the way back. I could hardly keep up with it."

I smiled at the image of a homesick mule running up a mountain pass. "The mule must have liked it on the farm. Did you like it there?"

"It was okay. It was home. But the work was hard. All day, every day, you work and work some more. Even the women work all the time. American's don't know about real work. You have it easy."

"Do you ever feel homesick?"

"What is 'homesick'?"

"Do you miss your old home? Do you miss Italy?"

"No. I don't miss anything. I know what's what. I know what you do. Why do you spy on me all the time? What do they do with all the blood they take from me? In Pittsburgh, I didn't go to the doctor all the time. Something's wrong. It don't make sense."

The time for pleasant reminiscence was over.

"You go the doctor more now because you had a heart attack. They check your blood to make sure it isn't too thick. That could cause another heart attack. Or if it's too thin, you could bleed inside and that would be very dangerous."

"Blood is blood. It doesn't get too thick or thin. Food doesn't go in your lungs. Something's wrong. It don't make sense. I'm going to tell the doctor you're keeping me upstairs all the time. That's enough bullshit for now. I need to sleep when I can. I don't sleep much."

I was dismissed.

Remembering the ringing phone, I checked the caller ID before getting into bed. It wasn't from Mike and I didn't recognize the area code, so I didn't bother listening to the message. It could wait until morning. I read for a couple of hours, keeping an eye out for activity in Rodger's room, but he was resting, quietly watching TV. I turned out the light, hoping he'd get a good night's sleep. I lay awake most of the night, listening to his breathing, just as I had when my children were babies.

I was puzzled by the message I found on the answering machine the next morning. Some of the words were too faint to understand, "… my name is … Someone you used to know loves you and misses you very much." Several seconds of silence followed and then, "Please call me at this number."

I jotted down the digits, not sure if I'd return the call or not. Who could it be? Was it a wrong number? If it was one of Mike's old girl friends, she was out of luck.

There was only one way to find out. I picked up the phone and placed the call. When a woman answered, I recognized the voice as the same one on the answering machine.

"Hello. Someone from this number left an odd message on my answering machine. Do you know what it's about?"

"Is your name Barbara Ann?"

"Yes. Do I know you?"

"Do you know Harry Simpson?"

I shivered as a combination of fear and anticipation raced through me.

"Hello? Are you still there?"

"Where is he?" I asked, pulling out a chair and sitting at the breakfast table. "Is my father alive?"

"He's alive and he's okay. I'm engaged to his son, Brian. They live together in Florida. He's been looking for you for a long time. When I was visiting them about a month ago, he asked me to go on the Internet and try to find you. I finally ran across your name and found a number. Before I tell you anything more, I want you to know that I care about him and I don't want to see him hurt. If you don't want to hear from him, I won't tell him I found you."

"Yes I want to hear from him." My voice was trembling. "He's the one who cut off contact. I wrote letters and sent cards for a long time but he never answered. He moved, but my address and phone number stayed the same for fifteen years. I never heard from him."

"All I know is he asked me to find you and I have."

"Can I speak to him?"

"He's not here. This is my cell number. I'll call him and tell him Brian will be contacting him in five minutes. Brian is a truck driver and is on the road. Pops will want to talk to him, so he'll be waiting by the phone. Here's the number."

I paced for five minutes, looking at my watch every few seconds. *She called him Pops. He always hated being called Pop. Maybe it isn't him after all. What if it is? Where has he been? What does he want? The message said someone you used to know loves you and misses you very much. Someone I used to know? You don't stop knowing your father. You may not see him for a long time, but you still know him. Is that how he feels? As if I'm some past acquaintance he'd like to touch base with?* I took a deep breath and waited for the last few seconds to tick by and reached for the phone again.

As soon as he said hello, I knew it was my father on the other end of the line. The protective shield I erected around my heart the day I realized he didn't want me anymore crumbled into dust. I loved him, no matter what.

"Hi, Daddy."

"Who is this?" he demanded, shock and suspicion clear in his voice.

"It's Bobbi," I answered, my voice shaking as hard as my hand gripping the phone.

"Bobbi? Is it really you? Baby, baby, baby. How did you get my number? Where are you?"

"I love you, Dad."

"Oh, Honey, I love you too."

I explained the mysterious phone call and how I'd spoken with Brian's fiancée who gave me his number.

We stayed on the phone for over an hour. He told me he was divorced from Brian's mother and explained how, after she left, he had found a large manila envelope full of photos, cards, and letters from me that he had never seen. I was shocked to learn of this betrayal. The first time I met my father's wife, she'd greeted me with a warm smile and a big hug. I couldn't imagine why she would have done such a cruel thing. I always hoped that if my father needed me, his wife would contact me.

I told him about his grandchildren and my life with Mike. The two men had spoken on the phone right after Mike and I were married, but they never met. I told him about my mother's death, the death of Mike's mother, and how Rodger now lived with us. When the call ended, I sat at the table trying to sort through the emotions sweeping through me. My joy at hearing my father's voice after more than twenty years was tainted with remembered pain and resentment. I believed his ex-wife had done what he said she did, and I hated the woman for it. But why didn't he call or write when he didn't hear from me? From what he said on the phone, I knew they had moved several times during those years—but I hadn't.

Oh ,Daddy, I thought. *I know you better now than I did then.*

The hero I saw through little-girl eyes never existed. The man who made me feel pretty as a teen when I cried after my mother pointed out how skinny I was turned his back on me and all his children when he divorced our mother. The man who should have been a grandfather to my children had missed everything by his own choice. But still I wanted him in my life. He had finally reached out to me, and I'd make the most of it.

He is flawed but so am I.

I couldn't wait to tell Mike the good news

Chapter 27

We were enjoying a drink before dinner at one of our favorite restaurants, thankful for the few hours of respite care that allowed us to spend time together every Saturday night.

I took another sip of wine and relaxed into the comfort of the well-padded booth.

"Happy?" Mike asked. He reached across the table for my hand. "I love you very much, and I'm so grateful for everything you do for me and my father. I'll do almost anything to see you smile."

"Yes I'm happy," I said. "I'm still more tired than I ever thought possible, even more than when the kids were babies, but in this moment, here with you, I'm very happy. And I can hardly wait until my dad gets here. I wonder how our fathers will get along."

Mike didn't say anything for a few minutes. I waited patiently for him to speak. I knew from the deep creases that formed above his brow when he was worried, that he was trying to find the right words to tell me something.

"What is it?"

"It's about this visit from your father." He sighed, hesitant to continue. "I've never met him, and he's going to be here for over a month. You never asked how I felt about all this. It's my house too. I'm not sure I want him here that long. What if I don't like him?"

I jerked my hand away. What the hell was he saying? How could he? How dare he?

"You think a month is too long to have my father in our home? I haven't seen him in over twenty years. He's old and not well, and this may be the only time I get to spend time with him. I can't go to see him because I can't leave your father, who I've been caring for day and night for six years, and you think a month is too much time for you to have to put up with my father?"

I couldn't stop the tears from streaming down my face. The waiter, who had come to ask if we were ready for another drink, took one look at me and scooted away as fast as he could. Pain and a sense of betrayal sliced through my belief in my husband, leaving only a tattered remnant in its place. I didn't know if I could bear the loss. Wounds as deep as that often fail to heal. I had never felt so alone. I was supposed to ask permission? Why? He shared my belief that family takes care of family. He knows how much I missed my father. For years I'd shared my hope of hearing from him again. I always thought he wanted that for me too. It never occurred to me that he'd try to keep my father from me.

Oh God, here it comes. My heart started pounding and I broke out in a cold sweat. I couldn't catch my breath. I stumbled in my haste to get out of the booth and into the ladies room before making an even bigger fool of myself in front of everyone in the restaurant.

The panic attack hit like a tsunami. Wave after wave of anxiety stripped away my defenses, leaving my nerves scraped raw by the sands of doubt. Where did I go wrong this time? How was it that no matter how hard I tried, someone found me lacking? The drink I savored just moments before burned its way out of me, leaving me weak and retching over the toilet.

When it finally passed, I soaked paper towels in cold water and bathed my face and neck. No one was going to take this opportunity from me! He was going to have to deal with my father. He didn't have a choice. My father was coming, he was going to stay at least a month, and I wouldn't listen to anymore crap about it.

When I returned to the table, our meals had arrived. We picked at our food in silence and went home. Mike never mentioned his reservations about the visit again. I did my best to hide my pain and anger and continued to make plans for my father's visit. I went through the intervening days in a haze of anticipation mingled with dread. What if Mike made his feelings known to my father? Would he leave early, never to be heard from again? Why had what should have been a happy reunion turned into another source of stress. The panic attacks continued, and every morning I scooped more hair off the shower floor.

"Nothing is ever easy," I said to my father a week before he was scheduled to arrive.

His breathing was raspy and labored over the phone. Over fifty years of smoking had left him with emphysema. He needed oxygen at all times. He'd need a wheelchair to take him to his plane and, upon arrival, to get him through the airport. I spent days trying to find a place willing to provide in-home oxygen on a temporary basis. The places I found were either unwilling to work with me, or didn't take my father's insurance. I even looked into buying a room air converter but it was far too expensive. He was getting frustrated and mentioned giving up on the idea of travel. I was afraid we'd have to put off the visit—then everything came together. His provider in Florida made arrangements with a provider near us, and in a matter of hours the problem was gone and his flight was booked.

The weather was cold and the ground covered with snow the evening we drove to the airport.

"I hope he thought to bring a warm coat," I said when we pulled into the short-term parking lot.

"Don't worry your pretty head. I grabbed one of Rodger's just in case," Mike said.

"Thank you. I can't believe I didn't think of it myself."

"You had a lot on your mind. You can't think of everything. Are you nervous?"

"Oh yes. Are you?"

"I'm okay. It's a little late for him to object to my marrying his little girl," he joked.

"And you're okay with his being here?"

"All I want is for you to be happy," Mike said, not really answering my question.

While we were waiting for my father to come off the plane, Mike got the portable oxygen tank ready—and I paced.

I wonder if I'll recognize him. Will he know me?

"There he is," Mike said.

I'd have known him anywhere, despite how much he'd changed. He'd always been extremely skinny. 'Not skinny, thin,' he'd insist when anyone commented on his appearance. At one hundred thirty-five pounds and six feet tall, he was skinny. I remembered my mother shocking me once by telling me she loved how he looked in a suit, hated how he looked naked. The last thing I wanted to picture as a teenager was my father naked. Age and illness had diminished him further. Even clothed he resembled a naked baby bird sitting in the nest of his wheelchair. I wondered if he was sicker than he let on.

"I made it," he said with a twinkle in his eye. "Come here and give me a kiss."

"You sure did," I said, moving toward him, my arms open for a hug I'd waited far too long to share with him.

The conversation on the way home was superficial and safe. Whenever my father spoke, Mike responded politely. "Yes, sir. No, sir. I'm glad you had a smooth flight, sir."

When we finally got home, it was late and he was clearly exhausted. I was afraid the ordeal had been too much for him. All he wanted to do was get to his room and go to bed.

"Oh my, that's a lot of stairs," he said when I explained the guest room was on the second floor. "My house in Florida is all on one floor."

"I'll help you and then I'll bring your luggage, sir." Mike said.

He turned and looked at Mike over the top of his glasses, a look that spoke of my childhood and all the times he'd looked at me or one of my siblings just like that. It was a signal that he was trying to hide his amusement by pretending to be stern.

"Listen, son, that's enough of the sir stuff. You can call me Harry. You can call me Dad. You can even call me Old Fart, but don't call me sir."

Mike didn't miss a beat. "My mother taught me to be respectful to my elders, but if that's the way you want it, okay. Where would you like me to put your suitcase, Old Fart, sir?"

My dad responded with a sigh and another look over the glasses at my wiseass husband, and I knew they were going to get along just fine.

With my father settled comfortably in his room, I checked on Rodger, who had watched the commotion of his arrival through a crack in his sitting room door.

"What's his name? How long will he be here?" he asked.

"His name is Harry, and he'll be here a month. He'll be here for Christmas and will go home right after New Year's."

"He's not going to live here?"

"No. He'll go back to Florida when it's time."

"Who takes care of him?"

"He lives with Brian, his stepson."

"Does he want him back?"

"Yes. You don't have to worry. He's not here forever."

"I don't worry. How long will he be here? I hope he doesn't eat all the pita bread."

"He won't," I assured him. I didn't bother reminding him that he didn't eat pita bread anymore.

"Goodnight, then. I hope he don't snore. I don't sleep much you know."

I said goodnight and joined Mike in our bedroom. "I can't believe how frail my father looks. I'm afraid for him. I hope I haven't killed him by bringing him here."

"I know!" Mike said, his eyes wide open in amazement. "There's nothing to him. I think his clothes weigh more than he does. I hope he's okay in the morning. I like the old fart."

"Thank God for that," I said.

"I'm sorry for what I said about his coming here. I didn't mean it the way it sounded. I had no idea what he'd be like. I didn't want you to be hurt by him again."

I accepted his apology; glad he was no longer opposed to my father's presence in our home. As I lay awake, listening for sounds from the old men in my care, I wondered if he understood how deeply he had hurt me.

By the time my father got up in the morning, Rodger had eaten his breakfast, had his medication, and was watching Bonanza reruns on TV. I was relieved to see that Harry looked much better. I'd never tell him that I had checked on him three times during the night to make sure he was breathing.

"The combination of the flight, and all the to-do about the oxygen, and being nervous about seeing you again, took a lot out of me but I'll be fine now. Don't worry."

I resisted the urge to tell him I never worried. He hadn't been here long enough to get the joke.

Rodger would be curious about our visitor, so after spending much of the morning talking with my father, still a bit dazed at seeing him sitting across the table from me drinking a cup of coffee, I helped Rodger down the stairs and left the two men alone while I went up to take a shower and get dressed. I already knew they'd be an interesting pair. Rodger, as diminished as he was, still bore some signs that for most of his life he had been a lot stronger than Harry. It was his mind that was deeply damaged. My father, slight all his life, and now a physical wreck, was as mentally sharp as ever. Between them, they could have made either one extremely healthy man or one travesty of a human being. I wondered how they'd interact during this visit, using their remaining combination of gifts and deficits to their advantage, and how I'd deal with it.

"I can go up the stairs better than your father," Rodger said one day.

"Yes you can," I agreed, allowing him a point of pride and not bothering to point out that he needed help to do it

"How old is he?"

"He's 82."

"He's older than me. Huh."

"Yes he is."

"When is he going home? Is he going to stay here? It's too much for you to take care of him. He takes food in the night. You didn't know that, did you? I hear him after you go to bed."

I reminded him that my father was leaving after the holidays, and reassured him that there was enough food for everybody, even if my father ate some during the night.

"You certainly have your hands full with him," my father said one afternoon as he watched me cook and puree lunch for Rodger. "Brian is at work all day, so I cook for myself when I'm home."

"Yes, you're much more capable of doing things like that. Even before his swallowing problem got this bad, I had to stop him from using the stove. He'd forget it was on and walk away. The combination of schizophrenia and dementia is awful."

Each man took pride in what they had left and ignored what they had lost, and I loved them both for that. I loved listening to them talk. Two o'clock had become Happy Hour for them. Every afternoon, I'd bring Rodger down and they'd sit at opposite ends of the table, drinking their beverage of choice, Ensure for one and Boost for the other, and talk about World War II, the Korean Conflict, and how much better things were in the old days. At night Mike would spend time with his father after dinner and then sit and talk and watch TV with Harry. Some days were good, and others were incredibly hard, depending on Rodger's mood, and if I was his friend or his enemy.

I spent hours talking with my dad. We reminisced about the happy times, and I questioned him about the time he was absent from my life. He still didn't own up to his responsibility for the long separation, but I no longer needed him to. I was grateful to have him back and cherished every moment.

We laughed, watching an old home movie that had been converted to a DVD. In it, my sister Kit was alive, still a child of ten. She and our cousin, Dee, were having a tea party outside. I was their maid, pouring water from an old coffeepot while they smoked stolen cigarettes. It was all a farce. Uncle Jim was filming it all, and it ended with Dad catching the wayward girls, taking off his belt, and giving my sister a very fake spanking.

Farther on in the film were scenes from a July Fourth picnic in the backyard. My grandparents and favorite aunts and uncles sat around the plank table, eating potato salad and hot dogs and drinking beer or Coke, while the cousins played in the background. My mother, six months pregnant with her youngest son, looked so young. It startled me when I did the calculation. My mother was thirty years old and carrying the fifth of her six children. *No wonder she lost patience with us so often,* I thought, *she was exhausted.* Feeling that way myself more often than not these days, I had a new understanding of my mother. We do the best we can under the circumstances. Sometimes we get it right and sometimes we make a royal mess of it, but we do it out of love.

Later that day I found my father sitting in the living room holding my mother's high school graduation picture. I keep it on display next to one of my father at the age of twenty. He looked at Mom with such love and longing it brought tears to my eyes. Despite the divorce and both of their remarriages, they shared an unbreakable bond. In that moment, I saw him fall in love with her all over again.

"She was a real beauty, wasn't she?" he said.

"Yes she was," I agreed.

"And I wasn't bad-looking myself, was I?"

"Not bad at all. You must have made quite a couple."

"We were so young. The times were so hard with the war and everything, but God how I loved her. I remember seeing her walking down the street with her schoolbooks in her arms and thinking, 'Now there's a girl!' She was the only one for me after that. We were married in church, you know, and Catholics don't recognize divorce. Despite what happened, she was always my wife, and I never stopped thinking about how I could have done things better."

I didn't know what to say, so I remained silent and joined him on the couch, slipping my arm around him. In the following days I often found him sitting quietly holding the picture. So I made a copy of it, and the one of him, and framed them as a Christmas gift. I liked the idea of my parents being together again.

Rodger was on his best behavior for most of the visit. He rarely accused me of keeping him prisoner, and only once did he insist that I was starving him to death. He kept a close eye on Harry and never failed to tell me if he did anything he considered wrong, including using too much toilet paper and staying up too late when we were out.

Mike and I spent a rare evening with friends, attending a Christmas party at a house nearby. When we got home, Harry was still up and Rodger was pacing in his room.

"I want you to know I was being babysat," Harry told us.

"What do you mean?" I asked.

"I was watching TV when Rodger came out of his room, pointed at his watch, and told me it was past 10:00 p.m. I told him I knew that, and he informed me it was time to go to my room. I told him I wasn't ready to go to bed yet, and he reminded me that you two were out and firmly told me to go to bed. I told him again I wasn't going, and he went back in his room in a huff. He's been checking on me every ten minutes since then."

"Well, we're going to bed, but you can stay up as long as you like," Mike told him ,shaking his head and laughing. "But don't go sneaking any girls in or you'll be grounded."

"Good night, Rodger," I called out as I passed his room. As soon as I spoke, his light went out and he didn't make a sound.

"What a pair," Mike said.

"Yes, Junior and Senior are something else," I answered.

When alone, we had sometimes referred to Rodger as "Junior" because of his childlike behavior, but calling Harry "Senior" was something new to Mike.

"It fits," I said. "My dad is older than yours, and his name is Harry Simpson, Senior."

"Okay, Junior and Senior it is. We have our own in-house comedy team."

"Speaking of an in-house team, what would you say to my dad coming to live with us?" I asked softly.

"If that's what you want, it's fine with me. It will be hard, but now that I've gotten to know him he's welcome anytime. Have you spoken to him about it, or has he said anything about wanting to come here?"

"No. I brought it up now because I need to know your feelings in case it comes up later."

"When or if it happens, you have my blessing."

"I'll need more than your blessing if it ever happens. I'll need your help, but your saying that means more to me than you know."

Christmas came and went in a flurry of visits from friends and family, and Harry got to meet two of his grown grandchildren and their families for the first time. It was awkward for them. His sudden appearance didn't warrant their immediate affection, but they were as welcoming to him as they would've been to any guest in our home. All in all, it went better than I expected. Rodger was very solicitous to Harry on Christmas Day, insisting he take the most comfortable chair and open his gifts first.

"You're the guest. You'll be leaving soon. I live here," he said several times during the day. I wondered if it was his subtle way of telling us all that he was ready for Harry to go home.

Two days before he was scheduled to leave, Senior surprised me by telling me he was reluctant to go.

"I'm an old man and I don't know how much longer the good Lord will keep me here on earth. I'd love to spend my last days here with you if it were possible. I want you to know that."

"It is possible if that's what you want. Mike and I talked about it, and he'd welcome you as much as I. Your room is ready now if you want to use it."

"I couldn't do it now. Brian was afraid if I came here I'd never go back. I promised him that wouldn't happen. You're my daughter, my flesh and blood, but he's my stepson, and I'd have been lost without him after his mother left us. I'd need time to break the news to him and prepare to leave, but the most important reason I can't do it is upstairs. You have your hands full with Mike's dad. I can't add to your burden."

"You're not a burden. You're my father and I love you. My home is your home if you decide this is where you want to be."

"I know and I wish it would work, but it's not fair to ask you to care for another old man."

Although I understood his words, in my heart what I heard was him choosing someone else over me. Again. I couldn't help wondering if, once he got back on the plane, I'd ever hear from him again.

Chapter 28

Everything quickly went back to normal after my father's visit. Rodger must have been exhausted from trying to outdo his rival. He paced and muttered for hours, day and night, and apparently I was to be punished for some reason. He didn't like the food, or I didn't give him enough. He didn't like my watching him, and he sure as hell didn't want to take his medication. He wanted to go downstairs on his own.

"It's okay if I try it two, three, four times a day. That's what the doctor meant. I have to go out sometimes."

"Let me know when you want to go out and I'll take you," I told him.

"You can't keep me up here. I'll tell the doctor. They don't know about you but I'll tell them. You're worse than Shirley. Worse than my mother."

"If you want to be down here, Mike and I will move your bed into the office and you can stay on the first floor. Would you like that?"

I asked him that every time he accused me of keeping him prisoner on the second floor. He said no every time; he didn't want his bed downstairs. He wanted to come and go as he pleased and that was far too dangerous. His doctors and nurses and home care providers all told him repeatedly that it was best for him to stay on one level. Despite all that, he was convinced I was the one pulling the strings. On bad days he was outright hostile. On good days he tolerated me, and on the rare very good day, he almost seemed to like me.

Every few days my father would call or I'd contact him. He sent cards and little gifts on occasion and I did the same for him. It was an imperfect relationship but a far better one than we'd had in years. I accepted it and appreciated every phone call and note.

I had just ended a call to him when movement on Rodger's monitor caught my attention. He shifted from one end of the couch to the other and cocked his head, as if listening for something, then he nodded, as if in agreement. Before going to his room to check, I watched him interact with his invisible visitor for a few more minutes, hoping I wasn't seeing what I knew was happening. The door was open but he hadn't heard me approaching. I stood transfixed as it became clear he was hearing voices again. The "others" had returned.

"Rodger, are you ready for a snack?" I asked, pretending I didn't know what was going on.

He didn't answer. I repeated my question a bit louder. That time I got through to him. He looked startled for a moment and then tried to pretend nothing had happened.

"Can I have some pudding?"

"Sure. Do you want chocolate or vanilla?"

"Vanilla. I can get it."

"No, you sit there and I'll be right back," I said.

"Don't tell me to sit! I sit when I want to sit. You're not the boss of me. I don't want your damned pudding. Go away. I can take care of myself!"

I didn't want a confrontation, so I left to get his pudding. I didn't take it right up to him; instead, I watched as the "others" regained his attention. I wondered who was there and what they were telling him. I hadn't seen any sign of the voices returning and was more than a little rattled to discover it now.

Once he stopped reacting to them and went back to watching TV, I took him his pudding and made sure he took small bites and swallowed three times before taking another spoonful. He glared at me and tried to scoop as much food onto the spoon as he could. Once, the look he gave me was so full of venom I barely recognized him. It was time to call Jackson and let him know what was going on.

He was as concerned by this latest development as I was. After conferring with Rodger's psychiatrist and his primary care doctor, Jackson called and told me a decision had been made to increase the dose of his Zyprexa and to add a prescription for a strong tranquilizer to be used as needed. He explained that after so many years on the medication, it could stop being effective. If that happened, Rodger would have to be admitted to long-term care facility for the mentally ill. In the meantime, they would hope the increase in antipsychotic medicine would work. If he became very agitated, I was to give him the Lorazepam right away. As hard as it would be to lose him, I prayed that if the medication stopped working, God would take him. Neither Mike nor I wanted to see him die in an institution. He had worked too hard and accomplished too much in his lifetime to end up that way.

Over the next year there were many more trips to the hospital. His C.O.P.D. worsened drastically, as did the dementia. He developed congestive heart failure, and despite the increase in medication, "the others" visited regularly. One day, when he was more lucid than he had been in long time, I asked him about the voices.

"Who are they?"

"They are who they are."

"What do they say to you?"

He refused to say. His only response was, "They make me feel nervous and suspicious."

I read that one of the reasons for his frustration and suspicion was that the voices often would be communicating with him while I was speaking, contradicting whatever I said or making it impossible for him to hear and understand me. The head of psychiatry at the hospital told me that the voices never say anything good. What he was hearing were vile accusations and humiliating insults about himself and the people around him. At times they whispered; other times, they screamed, day and night, disrupting his sleep and his every waking thought.

Often I had to reach for the Lorazepam in order to get some peace for him and for us. I rarely slept through the night anymore. Fatigue made it harder for me to cope with his ever-changing moods and verbal attacks. By the time Mike got home from work each day my stress level was soaring. We argued over little things and snapped at one another all the time. We were reaching a breaking point and we knew it. I called and requested respite care many times, only to be told that there were no beds available and respite care was on hold for the foreseeable future. They said if things were that bad I should look for a bed in a local nursing home. That would never work. Rodger wouldn't do well in a strange place. Even more important, his combination of ailments made it impossible to find a place nearby willing to take him. All I wanted was a few days off to rest and regain my mental and physical stamina. Things came to a head after Mike and I had a fight that left us both shaken. Lord only knows what started it, but I lost it and lit into him, accusing him of being insensitive to what I went through and accusing him of having it easy.

"*You* get up and leave for hours every morning. *You* spend the day with normal people. You have reasonable conversations and share jokes. *You* go out to lunch whenever you want. On the weekends you leave again and stay out most of the day running errands. Why don't you stay with him once in a while? Why don't you put up with his shit? Let him accuse you of starving him, even after you spend hours feeding him and he's signed for every bite of food I spent hours making for him. You stay awake all night listening for sounds of his footsteps, wondering if he's going to fall down the stairs and break his neck trying to get to food that will stick in his throat and make him cough and aspirate, then you sit with him for ten or twelve hours a day while he's in the hospital with pneumonia. My God, I'm here for him every day and all he does is bitch and complain. I take care of him and what thanks do I get for it? He's going to tell the doctor and his too-busy brother and his absent son how mistreated he is. Screw the whole damn bunch of you. I've had it!"

Mike stared at me in stunned silence. "You think this is easy for me? Yes I go to work every day. And I put up with all the crap that entails while I'm worried about what my father will do next. I worry about what it's doing to you and I wish to God I could do more to help, but I can't. There's only one of me. My job is to keep the bills paid and do the things that you can't do outside our home. I can't bear what this is doing to you. I see how tired you are. I see how nasty he can be to you.

"More than that, I see what you don't. I see that you make it harder on yourself than it has to be. You expect perfection, and when you can't attain it, you punish us both. What more do you expect from me? Jesus Christ, woman, if I offer to get up with him during the night, you tell me to go to sleep so I'll be able to go to work in the morning. If I offer to feed him, you hover over the monitor to make sure I'm doing it right. You want to leave the house but you're afraid that if you do something bad will happen that only you could have prevented. Stop trying to be a saint and stop being so damned hard on me! I need to get away from you for a while." He stalked away and up the stairs to our room, leaving me miserable and filled with new guilt. Everything he said was true, and I couldn't believe that I had caused him so much pain. He didn't deserve it.

Shit. Now what have I done? Why is it so hard to do good work, Lord? Can you tell me that? I had that question in my head almost all the time now. *Why does it have to be so hard?*

I got my answer the following Sunday. When the priest began to speak after reading the gospel, I felt that he was talking directly to me.

"I've been hearing the same question over and over lately. 'Why is life so hard? Why is it so difficult to do good works?' A chill ran through me. God had heard my cry.

"I'm here to tell you," the priest lectured, "no one ever told you it was supposed to be easy. In fact there are many examples in the Bible of people being tested to their very limits. It's in adversity that you grow in spirit. It's when you step up and do the hard stuff God asks of you that you earn your place in heaven. So quit whining and do what you know has to be done and remember you are not alone. He is there for you when you need Him."

After that, when things got very hard I tried to make light of it by telling Mike, "I earned my place in heaven today." He believed it, even when I didn't.

I was talking with Jackson one morning, going over Rodger's latest symptoms and medicine changes, when he asked how I was holding up.

"Not well. I've decided to call and ask for respite care again, and this time if they say no I'm calling my congressman. Rodger holds a 100% service-related disability rating, and he has the right to respite care so I stay in decent condition to do what's best for him. If that doesn't work, we're going to have to admit him to permanent long-term care. I can't go on like this without some kind of break."

"Do it," Jackson agreed. "Sometimes you have to demand what you need."

Two days later the patient advocate called to notify me that a bed would be available for Rodger the following Monday. They were approving six days of respite care. Within the hour I'd receive a request form, and all I had to do was fill it out and send it back as soon as possible. I said a silent prayer of thanks and called Mike.

"Find out if you can get some time off next week. Plan to sleep late and put your worries aside."

He called back fifteen minutes later to tell me he got the time off. We spent the six days catching up on sleep and relaxing at home. We enjoyed every minute of it.

Chapter 29

"I'm going back to Pittsburgh soon."

Rodger lay in a hospital bed, once again surrounded by old soldiers. I tried to tell the admitting physician that he should be in isolation because of his history with MRSA, but he didn't listen. All four beds in the ward were now filled and people were bustling in and out of the room, bringing breakfast, bathing patients, and delivering morning medication. I sat in a chair at the foot of his bed, despite the day nurse's protests. Visiting hours didn't start for another hour. I didn't care. I had to be there to make sure he received pureed food and to help him eat.

Months had passed since we had enjoyed our week off. Months where Rodger continued his steady decline. We doubted he'd see another New Year. Shortly after his return home that time, we began making funeral arrangements. Recalling the dreadful days after his mother's sudden passing, Mike wanted things in order long before they were needed. We had walked silently past the display of caskets, breathing in the awful scent of flowers and old perfume that permeated the place, remembering losses we'd already endured, dreading the agony to come. When the selection was finally made and the papers signed, we walked to the car in silence, hoping not to return anytime soon.

As much time as we spent together, Rodger still managed to surprise me. I smiled, remembering my last birthday. I recalled waiting for Mike to come to share a special dinner and watch as I opened my present. My gift, wrapped in paper suitable for a baby shower, was sitting on the kitchen table.

"It was either that or Christmas paper." Mike grinned when he placed it there the previous evening.

I loved the paper. Our daughter was expecting her first baby, and it was nice to be reminded of the joy to come.

It had been a busy morning. Rodger started pacing at 6:00 a.m. A dream, a memory, or something on the news made him anxious, and I knew well before taking his blood pressure that the reading would be high. The first reading was 190/100. After morning meds, it dropped a bit to 180/90. A half-hour later, his standing blood pressure held steady at 156/85. That was good enough. His heart was so damaged we aimed for acceptable, recognizing that optimum was no longer possible. The bronchitis that had plagued him for the past two weeks was finally gone.

Later in the morning I was surprised when the florist delivered a beautiful bouquet of spring flowers. The colorful mix of variegated tulips, yellow roses, day lilies, and hydrangeas was accented by sprigs of a purple flower I couldn't identify. It was from my daughter and son-in-law. The card read, "Happy Birthday, Momma. I love you."

"Happy birthday to you," Rodger sang when I showed him the flowers.

Touched, I took his hand in mine and thanked him. I didn't think he cared if it was my birthday.

"The flowers are very beautiful. Enjoy them while you can. You might be dead before your birthday comes again."

So much for a tender moment, I thought. But he was right, wasn't he? He reminded me to enjoy each day as it comes and that the future isn't guaranteed to anyone.

"Happy Birthday to me," I sang before taking a moment to heed his advice and stop and smell the flowers.

Rodger was thrilled when the baby came, a beautiful little girl named Ava. He loved to hold her and rock her. I had never seen such tenderness in his eyes. I knew I was watching something very special unfold when he looked at her. There was no fear or mistrust in him when he held such innocence. When her parents took her home, he'd sit in silence for the rest of the day, often holding her picture. He spent hours each day working on a latch hook rug for her, with me or the home health aide helping him grasp the yarn. I hoped he'd finish it before he became too weak to continue. I wanted to take a picture of the two of them so Ava would always have it to remember him.

"I'm going back to Pittsburgh soon," Rodger repeated, pulling me out of my reverie.

It's the dementia talking, I thought—until he spoke again.

"I'll be with Shirley again. There's room for me right beside her. Michael promised to take me back."

Don't cry. Don't say a word, just listen. I fought back the tears and tried to swallow the lump in my throat. I sat perfectly still, knowing at this moment he trusted me more than anyone.

"I had a dream last night. God told me my job here is done. Michael promised to take me back."

"Yes, when the time comes, Michael will make sure you go back to Pittsburgh. We don't know when that will be, but I promise you we will take you home."

He looked at me for several long moments before nodding his head and drifting off to sleep. I sat quietly, tears streaming down my face. I knew that the message he received in his dream was real, and I thanked God for assuring him that when his time came he could leave without regret. When I knew he was sleeping soundly, I gathered my things and was about to leave in search of a priest when a nurse came in and announced they were moving him to a private room.

"He's supposed to be in isolation," she said.

I agreed and stepped out after getting directions to the chapel.

The priest wasn't in the office when I arrived. I was greeted by the Protestant chaplain who invited me to sit with him and asked the secretary to page the priest. He was such a kind man that while I waited I had no trouble sharing what had happened. Eventually, both clergymen sat with me and asked questions, wanting to learn about Rodger and his life. They were surprised to find out that Rodger was my father-in-law and Mike's stepfather.

"Amazing. So many of our patients never see their family. and here you are taking care of someone who isn't a blood relative to either of you. He is blessed to have you both," the chaplain said.

The priest nodded his agreement. "You will be rewarded in heaven for your love and kindness."

"I'm not so sure about that," I said. "I make so many mistakes with him. I lose my temper and shout at him sometimes. It's so much harder than I ever thought it would be. Sometimes I resent him and wish it could be over so I can have my life back. I'm not so saintly after all, am I?"

"If you recall, the saints never had an easy time of it, but they believed in God and they continued their work."

"I'm no saint," I insisted. "I'm as flawed a woman as they come, and Rodger knows it better than anyone."

"And yet he trusts you," the priest replied. "He shared his message from God. Perhaps there was some wisdom for you in there as well?"

When it was time to leave, they assured me they would pray for Rodger and for me and Mike. Before going to Rodger's new room, I called Mike and told him what his father had said. He was sad but not surprised. He reminded me that no one knew how much time he actually had left.

"He's rallied many times before, so don't be surprised if he does it again."

I agreed, but deep in my heart I knew this time was different.

Chapter 30

Rodger was still asleep when I arrived in his new room, and he stayed asleep through lunch and dinner. The nurses assured me he was all right, just exhausted from fighting his illness and being jostled around so much.

"Go home. He's safe with us. If anything changes, someone will call you."

He was sleeping again when I got there in the morning. The nurse at the desk said he'd had a very quiet night. I arrived there early, before his breakfast tray was delivered, and it was a good thing I did. It was a standard breakfast. When I told the porter Rodger couldn't eat it and required a special diet, he said there was no notation about it on the menu form.

"This happens a lot, and it shouldn't," he said. "I'll take this away and ask his nurse to order the right meal. But it may take awhile to get things sorted out."

"That's okay. He's still asleep so we can wait. Thank you for your help."

While I was waiting, I dumped the cup of ice water sitting on his bedside table and threw the straw in the trash. Then I went to the commissary and bought a pad of paper, a marker, and tape. When the doctor came by on rounds, he found me busy posting signs all around Rodger's bed, again reminding his nurses not give him a razor or water or straws or solid food. I didn't bother getting angry this time. I was too damned tired to fight. I'd watch over him and keep him safe.

After a quick check of his vital signs, the doctor made some notes in his chart and left me to my work while he moved on to his next patient.

The replacement breakfast came and went and so did his lunch, and still Rodger slept. Every now and then, his eyes would open for a few seconds and he'd look at me and nod before drifting off again.

Late in the afternoon he was hooked up to an IV to keep him from becoming dehydrated. Both the priest and the chaplain stopped by to see him and offer prayers. Jackson sat with me for a while and assured me he was talking with the staff to make sure they were aware of Rodger's special needs and to make sure I'd be allowed to stay with him at all times.

"I told them you are as informed as any nurse about his needs, and they should be thankful you're taking some of the burden off them. The good ones agreed."

"And the not-so-good ones?"

"Screw them. And don't tell anyone I said that."

"I won't. I need you too much to risk your getting fired."

Rodger remained in a deep sleep for three days. He slept through mealtimes and bed baths and changes to his linens. Mike and our daughter and son-in-law came to sit by his side. Nurses and aides looked in with sympathy when passing his room. I only left his side to make calls or go to the commissary for a quick snack. I prayed each night when I left that he'd still be alive in the morning. I didn't want him to die alone.

I was shocked on the morning of the fourth day to find him sitting up in bed, waiting for his breakfast.

"I'm hungry," he said when he saw me. "I have to eat sometime."

"Yes you do," I agreed. "How long has he been awake?" I asked when a nurse came in to check on him.

"They told me he woke up around 2:00 this morning. He took out his IV and wandered into the hall asking for you. You're his daughter, right?"

Before I could answer, the nurse continued. "They had to move his bed out to the nurse's station to keep an eye on him. Even after they put the alarm on his bed, he refused to stay put."

"He's doing much better then?"

"He's very weak, and there's still a lot of fluid in his lungs. The doctor can tell you more when he comes in, but he shouldn't be walking around. After he eats, we can try letting him sit in a chair for a while but that's it."

When his breakfast came, I did my best to help him eat but he had difficulty swallowing even tiny amounts. His thickened juice didn't go down any better. Before long he gave up. The same thing happened at lunch. I managed to get a few bites of mashed potato and some pureed peas into him before he pushed the tray aside in frustration. When the doctor came in late in the afternoon, he took me aside and confirmed what the nurse had said, the pneumonia was not responding to treatment. He ordered a second medication to be added to his IV and requested another test to get an up-to-date reading on his dysphasia. In the meantime, a nasogastric tube would be inserted to get some nutrients into him.

I stayed at his side throughout the day and long into the evening. When I finally made it home, I wanted nothing more than a hot meal and a warm bed. Mike was in our home office. I went in to give him a kiss and an update on Rodger's condition.

When I finished, he hugged me and asked, "What's for dinner?"

"I don't know. You can cook it, you can go get it, you can place an order for delivery, but it's not up to me tonight. Right now, I need a hot shower."

I stood under the hot water, wondering how he could have asked that question. He was home all afternoon, having taken time off to work on updating the software on our computer. He had plenty of time to make dinner. I didn't care what it was, as long as I didn't have to decide.

When the water began to run cold, I turned off the shower, donned my robe, wrapped my wet hair in a towel, and went downstairs to make a cup of tea. Mike stood in front of the open refrigerator, searching for something.

"What do you want to eat?" he asked.

"I don't care. Pick something."

He closed the refrigerator and opened the freezer. "We have some hot dogs."

When I didn't say anything, he closed the freezer door and said, "I take that as a no. Okay, how about some pasta?"

"That's fine." I was rapidly losing patience with all the questions. Did he not hear me?

He opened the freezer again. "I can thaw some ground beef if you want a cheeseburger, but you probably don't want to wait for it to thaw in the microwave before I can cook it."

"Damn it! I don't believe you. Make a freaking decision. Cook or order something. I told you it's not up to me tonight! What the hell is wrong with you? Can't you see I don't have anything left to give right now?"

I stormed out of the kitchen and up the stairs to the bedroom. The echo of the slamming door reverberated throughout the house, followed by the sound of crying as I lost the tenuous control I had been holding onto all day. All I wanted was something to eat and someone to care enough about me to provide it. Even as I sobbed my heart out, I waited to hear the sound of cooking, or Mike's voice placing an order for pizza, or for him to come up and comfort me. When none of that happened, I wallowed in self-pity until that abated, then I got mad all over again. I wiped my eyes, blew my nose, and went looking for my husband. I found him, once again, in front of the computer.

"So you have no intention of taking care of dinner?" I accused.

"I would if you'd simply tell me what the hell it is you want!"

"I keep telling you what I want. I want you to do it. I have been at the hospital all day and most of the evening. I'm tired and I'm hungry. Why can't you do that for me? Why didn't you think about this long before I got home? You were here. You know where the food is. You know how to use the stove."

"I can't talk to you when you're like this," he snapped.

"I wasn't like this until you refused to listen when I asked you over and over to take care of dinner. You know damned well if the situation were reversed, if you had spent the day at the hospital and

I was home all afternoon, that there would be a meal waiting for you when you got home. So why didn't you do something? Why don't you care enough to do that for me?"

"I do care and you know it! I didn't do anything wrong and you come in here yelling at me for no reason."

"You have a piss-poor way of showing it today. I didn't start yelling until you refused to hear me when I said many times that I was not responsible for dinner. I didn't even tell you to cook it. But no, you kept pushing the decision back on me. And when you saw how upset I was, you still did nothing. You're still doing nothing."

With a heavy sigh, Mike rose from the computer and went to the kitchen, nuked some ground beef to thaw it, and made some cheeseburgers.

I was tempted to hit him for that sigh. He had no right to feel sorry for himself. But I didn't. I ate in silence, prayed for the day to end, then went to bed, hoping the morning would take a long time to arrive. I fell asleep almost immediately but awoke with a start two hours later to find Mike cradling me in his sleep.

When I stirred, he pulled me closer and whispered, "I love you."

I regretted the way the day had ended and wished I had handled it better. Remembering my thoughts about hitting him, I knew I'd never actually do it, no matter how dense his behavior. I smiled and snuggled closer to him, recalling a time when he was just as frustrated with me.

It happened before we were married, during the time his mother was determined to split us up. When she found out I planned to attend an out-of-town event with him, she decided to go herself. Knowing what a disaster that would be, Mike asked me to stay home. His mother was a friend of the hosts of the party, so it made sense that she be there. Neither of us wanted to give in, leaving him stuck in the middle. He kept asking me to be the bigger person and let this one thing go.

When I refused, he said, "You make me so I mad I want to throw socks at you!"

It was only as I lay in his arms that night that I truly understood the love in that statement. "I'm angry and frustrated as hell and I want you to know it, but I will never hurt you."

"I love you too," I murmured to his sleeping form. "But you should have taken care of dinner."

Chapter 31

"He had another bad night," the nurse said the next morning.

"I'm not surprised. He suffers from sundowning and has a bad night more often than not."

When it first started happening I learned "sundowning" is the term used to refer to confusion that occurs at the end of the day and into the night in people with dementia.

"Well, he sure had it last night. He ripped out his catheter and his IV and set off his bed alarm so many times they had to assign an aide to sit with him. Even moving his bed out to the nurse's station didn't help. He kept asking for you. He said you know what's what."

"He's sleeping now," I said. "I peeked in on him. He must have worn himself out."

"Himself and the entire night staff," the nurse agreed. "By the way, someone will be in to see you later to go over the results of his swallowing test."

"Not good?"

"I don't think so, but let's wait for the official results before we jump to conclusions."

When Rodger woke up, I filled a plastic basin with warm water and handed him a soapy washcloth to bathe his face and neck. He liked doing it for himself. Then I gave him his comb and watched as he ran it through his hair. The end result was the same as when he started.

"You're looking good this morning," I lied.

"Yeah, a lot of girls wanted to dance with me. My mother wanted me to get married but I didn't have time for that. Not until Shirley. She wanted to marry me. I raised those two boys. That's what mattered."

I agreed and was trying to get some pudding into him when the throat specialist arrived.

"His dysphagia has increased significantly, making it harder than ever for him to get adequate nutrition. I suggest you consider having a feeding tube put in place. The nasal tube he has now is only a temporary measure and can't stay in place much longer."

"Tell me about the feeding tube. How is it put in and what are the risks and benefits? I'll need to know how to care for it as well."

After hearing about the surgery he'd need and the risk of infection after it was inserted, I wanted to talk to Jackson before telling Mike about this latest development. Once Rodger was settled, I went to Jackson's office to see if he had time for me.

"Come in. I was planning to come and see you," Jackson said when he saw me standing in the outer office. "I hear our guy is having a hard time."

"He is and I need some advice. The throat specialist wants us to consider a feeding tube, and I'm not sure it's a good choice for him. What do you think?"

"Before I weigh in, what are your thoughts?"

"Like many schizophrenics, he tracks what goes into and out of his body. Having another device implanted will really upset him. He's deeply suspicious of all of us right now. I hear him mumbling about the box in his chest, and several times he's asked me where the wires go. Every week, when blood is drawn for his clotting test, he asks me what the government is doing with it. Lord only knows what he'll do when he sees me putting something into him three times a day."

"You're right. He'll fiddle with it and pull it out. You can bank on that. Truthfully, patients like him don't do much better with it than without it. It's your decision, but I don't think it will help him."

"Thank you for hearing me out. I'll talk this over with Mike and when we decide I'll let you know."

I rose to go but Jackson waved me back into my chair.

"I think it's time to apply for hospice. You know there's a facility right here that he's entitled to use. The doctors and nurses are wonderful. He'd be evaluated, and if accepted as a patient, he'd be given palliative care to keep him comfortable and pain free. But the weekly needle sticks and other invasive treatments will stop."

I knew this day would come, but I was still uncomfortable talking about it.

"He said more than once that he wants to die at home."

"There's also an in-home hospice program available. There are only ten beds in our unit. There isn't always one available, but he'd be given priority if one is open. If you'd like, I can call down there and find out if we can come by so you can learn more about it."

I agreed and Jackson made the call. An hour later I had talked to an admissions person and been given a lot of printed material to share with Mike later. My thoughts were going in several different directions when I got back to Rodger's room, where I found a nurse helping him back into bed.

"As soon as you left the room, he pulled out his IV and catheter again and got up, setting off the alarm. He was about to fall when I came in. It's lucky I got to him in time."

"Even if I fall, it won't be that bad. You worry too much, like her," he told the nurse.

"I was talking to the hospice coordinator. She gave me these pamphlets to go over with my husband."

The nurse looked at me, nodded in understanding, then returned to getting Rodger safely tucked into bed. Exhausted from his latest escapade, he drifted off almost immediately and slept through most of the afternoon.

"You still here?" he said when he awoke.

"I'm still here." I smiled at him.

"Go home. Don't worry about me."

"I'm not worried, but there's no one at home to talk to. I'll stay here until after you have dinner. Then I'll go."

"Do what you want," he sighed.

At change of shift, when a new nurse came in and introduced herself, Rodger said, "Pleased to meet you. When am I going to die? Will it be today?" he looked at his watch. "How much time do I have?"

"Only God knows that," the nurse answered with no hesitation. "And he didn't put an expiration date on your foot, so you should do what you can to get better and go home."

"Home sweet home," he said. And with those words, he confirmed my belief that in-home hospice would be the right choice for him. I hoped Mike would agree.

All the way home I thought about the decisions we'd have to make and how it would affect Mike. Deciding to pass on the feeding tube could appear to some people as agreeing to let him starve to death, something Rodger often accused me of doing. Would hospice care, either in the hospital or at home, send a message to others that we were willing to stand by and let him die?

I was so deep in thought that I drove for miles on autopilot. At one point I came to a stoplight and looked around, wondering where I was and how I got there. Had I passed my turnoff or was it still somewhere up ahead? Nothing looked familiar and I feared I had lost my way. After several moments of panic, I decided to continue on rather than take a chance on making a wrong turn. I began to recognize the landscape several miles down the road. I was on the right path after all. Was the slip-up meant as a message for me? Was I to continue on as I'd been doing and follow my instincts? Was it possible that I did know what I was doing after all?

Who the hell knows, I thought.

When I finally made it home, Mike was waiting for me with a cup of tea and a warm hug. He took my hand and led me to the table and set a plate in front of me. When I looked at the wonderful meal, I got up and hugged and kissed him again.

"Thank you. This looks delicious."

"It should. The Colonel spent all day cooking it for you," Mike joked.

I ate every bite of the baked chicken, mashed potatoes, and green beans as he looked on. I knew it was his way of apologizing for the misunderstanding the day before, and although his lapse still rankled, I was so grateful for the hot meal, I'd never let on.

"You and the Colonel make a good team and I do appreciate it."

"I'm sorry about last night," Mike said.

"Me too."

"I feel bad that you have to deal with all this."

"Don't," I said. "I do this, as hard as it is, because I care about him. What I'll need is time to recover. When this is over, and after we've had time to grieve, I want to go away for a while. I want a month off. I don't care where we go or what we do. It can be down the road to the local no-tell motel or a trip anywhere in the world, as long as I can sleep as late as I want, eat when I feel like it, and don't have schedules to keep."

"I'll make it happen," Mike promised. "But for right now, you look beat."

"I am. It's been another long day, and there are some things we have to talk about, decisions to be made."

"That sounds ominous."

"I'm afraid it is."

I told Mike about the throat specialist's recommendation for a feeding tube and my talk with Jackson. I was relieved when Mike agreed immediately that it would be better for his father to pass on that. We spent the rest of the evening reading and sharing the information about hospice care. After going over all of it, we agreed to schedule a tour of the hospital unit and learn more about the in-house option.

We were impressed with the hospice facility and the people who take care of the patients. We were grateful it was available for those who needed it. However, we knew before the tour was over that Rodger would not be staying there.

"He told me many times that when the time comes he wants to die at home. If you can provide help that allows us to give him that gift, we want to do it," I said and Mike agreed.

"You have so few beds and so many needy veterans. Keeping Rodger with us will give him what he wants and allow you to take care of someone else."

"Thank you for stepping up and taking such good care of him," our guide said. "He's been approved for in-home hospice care already, but it will take several days to make arrangements for everything you'll need. In the meantime, we can discharge him from the hospital. You'll probably be able to take him home sometime tomorrow. A hospice care supervising nurse will call in a day or two and schedule a time to come out, along with a social worker, to go over everything again and assess your home for safety and determine what equipment you'll need.

"Once he's in care, he won't have blood draws or any invasive treatment. You'll need a DNR (do not resuscitate) certificate certified by his doctor. Tape it to your refrigerator so it's readily available at all times. Believe me, you don't want emergency medical personnel doing CPR on him. It's brutal and not very effective in a case like his. In fact, as frail as he is, it could kill him. But without that certificate, no matter what you say, they're required by law to do it. Good luck to you and your loved one."

The next day Rodger was discharged, and he and I left the VA hospital for the last time.

Chapter 32

Before leaving, I stopped by Jackson's office to return the telehealth monitor that had connected us for so long. I thanked him for his devotion to helping others, for the long hours he spent researching the myriad of symptoms afflicting Rodger, and working so hard to get his doctors to pay attention when they dismissed my instincts. He had been my lifeline, as well as Rodger's, always insisting I had far more ability than I realized.

"You may not have a degree but you're a nurse. When the time comes that I need help, I want you to be the one taking care of me. Tell Rodger I wish him the best."

Before he had a chance to say more, he was called to the phone. Another caregiver needed him.

I wasn't prepared for the wave of emotion that swept over me as I passed the guard shack and turned for home. I had driven the many miles to this place and back so many times in the past six and half years I didn't doubt my car knew the way on its own. The people there were as familiar to me as my neighbors: The guards who greeted us each time we entered the building, the people who manned the canteen who came to know Rodger's favorite foods, the long-term patients who walked or wheeled themselves through the halls, my favorite pharmacist who always greeted us with a smile no matter how busy he was, and remained infinitely patient with my questions when a new medication was added.

I had observed the seasons pass in those halls. President's Day banners made way for St. Patrick's Day decorations that were taken down and replaced by Easter greetings. All through the year they made an effort to brighten the spirits of those who came and went, ending with a gaily decorated Christmas tree before starting over in the New Year. In all that time I had encountered far more nurses, doctors, and aides who did everything possible to make sure the sick, wounded, and elderly patients were treated with care and respect than those few who appeared to have lost heart and were there only to do a job.

How will Rodger cope with all these changes, and how can I go on without their help?

"When do we have to come back again?" Rodger asked.

I was startled by his words. We were almost home and it was the first time he'd spoken. I thought he was asleep.

"You don't have to go back anymore. If you need a doctor, one will come to the house. And you don't need to have blood tests anymore. You don't have to have the breathing treatments three times a day either. Isn't that good news?"

"How come? It don't make sense."

"The hospital is full, so they're sending a new bed and some other equipment to help me take care of you. They have a program to help keep patients at home whenever possible."

"Too many patients from too many wars," he said.

"Yes," I agreed.

"You have to tell me the truth. Don't hide what the doctors say."

"I won't. You have the right to know. I will never lie to you and you're always in the room when I talk to the doctors. You can ask questions anytime. Is there something worrying you?"

"When am I going to die?"

"We don't know. It could be a long time. It could be soon. If I know, I'll tell you. Right now we're getting things ready for when it comes. Nurses will visit every week to check on you. We'll make sure you don't have pain. Don't worry, Mike and I will be with you."

"I don't worry about nothing. When do we have to go back?"

I was grateful Rodger had come home on a Friday. We could use the time before the hospice coordinator arrived on Monday to plan where all the equipment would go and rearrange Rodger's room.

We were sitting at the kitchen table and Mike was sketching options for equipment placement when the phone rang.

"It's for you. It's Brian and he sounds upset," Mike said.

I felt the blood drain from my face. I didn't want to take the call. I didn't want to hear what I feared he would say.

"Bobbi, it's Pops." His voice was thick with unshed tears.

"Tell me." My voice was barely above a whisper.

"He's in the emergency room and it doesn't look good. The doctor can't believe he's still breathing."

"But he is alive?" I asked.

"For now, yes."

"What happened?"

"He hasn't been feeling well for a few days. I asked him if he wanted to go to the doctor and he said no. He hasn't eaten or slept much either. He insisted he wanted to be left alone. Then he woke me at 4:00 a.m. and said he felt worse. Tammy was here and she told him she was calling an ambulance. He didn't want to go but she called anyway. He's going to be mad about that. But I didn't do it, she did."

I was furious hearing that but tamped down my anger. This was not the time to address what I saw as negligence.

"Tell me exactly what the doctor said."

"His blood oxygen was very low. He has a low-grade fever too. The doctor said his lungs are so full of holes it's a miracle he's alive. They're moving him to ICU now and told us to contact any family and let them know."

I heard a voice in the background calling Brian.

"The doctor has some questions for me. I have to go. I'll call you back after I talk to him." He hung up, leaving me pale and shaking, holding the phone.

"What is it?" Mike asked.

"My father. He's dying." I doubled over in grief, racking sobs tearing through me. "I can't do this. It hurts too much. God help me, I can't. I can't!"

"I wish I could fix this and lift this burden from you." Mike's eyes filled with tears as he eased me up from the chair and into his arms.

"What's wrong with her?" Rodger called from the top of the

stairs.

"It's her father," Mike answered.

"Is he dead?"

"No, but he's very sick and he may not make it."

"Everybody has to die sometime. It's no use crying about it." And with that he turned his walker around and went back to his room.

Now it was my turn to pace. Every minute, for over two hours, the fear and tension grew. I wanted to speed to the airport and get on the first plane to Florida. I had to go to him. I had to save him. But I couldn't bear the idea of being in midflight when he passed away.

"I want to throttle Brian," I said when I could finally speak. "Why on earth would he ask Dad if he wanted to go to the doctor? How could he stand by and let him get worse? You don't ask him. You tell him. You pick up the phone and you call an ambulance. Jesus Christ, he's an idiot."

The phone rang, interrupting my tirade. I grabbed it, needing to know something, terrified by what he'd say.

"He's going to be all right," Brian said. "They're going to release him in the morning."

I nearly passed out from relief and shock. "What do you mean? How could he improve so much so fast?"

"The ICU doctor looked at his x-rays and said the ER doctor read them wrong. They show his emphysema is progressing, but he's not in danger of dying today. He's dehydrated, so they're keeping him on an IV overnight and releasing him in the morning. I have to go now. They're moving him to a regular room and he's calling me."

"Keep me posted if anything changes and call me when he gets home tomorrow so I can talk to him."

"I will." And he was gone.

"What did he say?" Mike asked.

"He said my father is going home tomorrow." I shared everything Brian had told me, and the two of us sank in relief into the nearest chairs.

"How could he put you through that, not knowing the details?" Mike asked, fury blazing in his eyes.

"He's an incompetent idiot who's going to stand by and let my father die because he doesn't have the balls to stand up to a sick old man—and there's nothing I can do about it."

"I wish I could do something to make it better," Mike said.

"Me too. For now I need a hug and a hot shower, and after that I need a drink. Forget I ever said anything about not drinking under stress. And by the way, I earned my place in heaven the last few days."

Chapter 33

My hands were slick with sweat when I greeted the hospice case manager and the social worker assigned to us. Rodger had picked up on my anxiety. I watched him via the monitor on the kitchen counter while the two women took seats and arranged piles of paperwork on the table. Every few seconds, he shifted from one end of the couch to the other, nodding or shaking his head. He seemed to shrink before my eyes in response to whatever hell the voices of the "others" were visiting upon him.

"Don't be nervous," the case manager said. "I know this is a very hard time for your family, and all this paperwork looks intimidating, but I'll do most of the work and spend as much time with you as you need while I explain how this works. And don't assume just because we're here that he's going to die soon. Some very sick patients move out of hospice care and spend a lot of quality time with their families. Some recover completely."

I sensed Rodger wouldn't be one of them, and I suspected the caseworker felt that way too.

"Is he up there alone? How do you know if he needs you when you're down here?" the social worker asked.

Her mouth opened in surprise when I pointed to the monitor and explained I carried it with me from room to room as I went about my day. Later it sat on my bedside table and I checked it frequently through the night.

Before starting on the paperwork, they asked to tour the house. They were pleased that Rodger had his own rooms all on one floor. They planned what equipment would be needed and where it would go. They spent time talking to Rodger, explaining about the new bed he'd be getting, and how he didn't have to go to the hospital to see his doctors anymore. When needed, the doctor would come to him. He was very happy to hear from them that the weekly needle sticks to draw blood were over. He had forgotten that I had already told him that.

"They got all the information they need already," he said. "The government is everywhere. They know all about you. They even know I'm going to die. That's why you're here."

"Mr. Carducci, you look pretty good to me," the caseworker replied. "Our job is to keep you comfortable and safe. The dying part is up to God, and he didn't share that information with any of us."

"Yeah, yeah," he answered, waving them off. "Nobody knows what God and the government knows. That's enough, you can go now."

Once the paperwork was signed, the caseworker started making calls. She ordered a hospital bed with an alternating pressure mattress pad to prevent bedsores, a rolling tray table, and a bedside commode.

"I don't want him walking to the bathroom all the time. Short walks down the hall are okay, as long as someone is with him and he uses his walker. If he falls, call the emergency number I'm going to give you before I leave. The last thing we want is for him to break a hip. Even if he insists he's okay, call and report it. He could have internal bleeding."

I promised to do everything they recommended.

"I'm also ordering a comfort kit. It will include a number of medications to use as needed. Keep it in the refrigerator. I hope you don't ever have to open it, but it will be there if you do."

"What's in it?"

"Liquid morphine you'll use for pain and shortness of breath. There's also a morphine suppository in case he can't swallow the liquid. He has emphysema and you don't want him to die gasping for breath. In addition to that, there's a liquid anxiety medicine, Atropine, to treat wet respirations, sometimes called a death rattle, Haldol for agitation or restlessness, Phenergan to treat nausea and vomiting, and rectal suppositories to treat constipation."

"Morphine?" I was shocked.

"This is medical-grade morphine. It's nothing like the stuff sold on the streets. His doctor ordered it to make sure he remains comfortable and pain free. Don't hesitate to use it when he needs it."

"What if I give him too much?"

"It's impossible for you to give him an overdose. Give him as much as he needs to keep him comfortable. I'm going to call and order the kit to be delivered right away." She picked up her phone and made the call. I was shaken when I heard the one-sided conversation. The caseworker identified herself and provided an ID number then said, "Please expedite it. I have a bad feeling about this one."

"Do you really think it's urgent?" I asked when the call ended.

"I do. Despite how well he seems to be doing, I've seen enough cases to be concerned. He could go either way and I want to be ready. Expect to hear from the nurse assigned to his care later in the day. She'll be calling to arrange for her first visit and plan a schedule for the weeks to come. Probably twice a week to start. You'll have her cell phone number to call if you need help during the day, and another number to call during the night. Someone would be available at all times."

"They still here?" Rodger called out.

"Still here, Mr. Carducci, but I'm leaving soon," the caseworker answered.

"Good!" he answered. The women laughed when he made a rude gesture on the monitor to punctuate his comment.

A few minutes later the case manager and social worker were gone. After seeing them out, I taped the glaring yellow DNR form to the front of the refrigerator and rearranged things inside to make room for the comfort kit.

"If that doesn't ruin one's appetite, I don't know what will," I said to myself as I went up the stairs to check on Rodger.

"Who were you talking to?" he asked, startling me.

Despite all the warnings he'd just heard from the caseworker, he was out of his room without his walker.

"No one," I answered. I took his arm and led him back to the couch.

"People say I'm crazy. You talk to yourself. You're the crazy one."

"I think we're both a little crazy. That's why we get along so well."

"Yes we get along. When am I going to die? All these people come but they don't tell me anything."

"I'll always tell you the truth," I promised. "I don't know when you will die. But I promise you this, I'll do everything I can to be with you and make sure you don't have pain."

"I'm not afraid to die. Living is the hard part. I did a good job. Everyone has a destiny. Don't tell Michael I'm dying. He's not ready."

By the time his new bed and the other equipment were scheduled to arrive, we had removed the old couch and rearranged the room to accommodate them. Once everything was in place, with the bed tight up against the wall on one side, I was happy to see that his recliner still fit. Each day I helped him into it and changed his sheets. If he wasn't to have a shower that day, I brought in a basin of warm water and washed him. If he felt up to it, I sat and watched TV with him until lunchtime. Then he was ready for a nap.

For several weeks, Rodger continued to do well. His nurse came twice a week, and a nursing assistant came once a week to help him shower. He enjoyed their company and they enjoyed his. I was beginning to believe he'd no longer need hospice care, when he began a slow but steady decline. He ate less and slept more. He no longer protested using the bedside toilet. He lost interest in his favorite TV programs. Only when baby Ava came to visit did he show any interest in what was going on around him. Upon seeing her, a light shone in his eyes. As little as she was, she seemed to sense he loved her, and she responded to him by cooing and laughing and touching his face. It was wonderful to watch.

The nights were the hardest. Every evening at sundown he became agitated and restless. He accused me of keeping him prisoner, and often recoiled at my touch when I tried to calm him. More and more often, I had to feed him Lorazepam-spiked applesauce to keep him safe.

Everyone told him not to get out of bed on his own. He was far too unsteady and a fall could be fatal. When he refused to listen, I started putting the side rail up on the bed whenever I left the room. It didn't take him long to discover he could get out through the gap in the rail and the foot of the bed. He called it his shortcut. He fell twice, scaring me. I had to place an emergency call to his nurse to come and check him for internal bleeding or broken bones.

After the second fall, a bed alarm was ordered to alert me when he was trying to get up. I also started placing the rolling tray table in the gap, blocking his shortcut. An intercom was on at all times so all he had to do was call to me and I'd go to him. Within days he was pushing the tray table out of the way and putting himself in danger again. He was setting off the bed alarm constantly. I took to sitting at his side all day, ready to help him into the chair or to the toilet. He hated all of it. It pained me to see him so unhappy.

Nights were even worse. Short naps during the day meant he was awake at all hours. I was awake too, keeping an eye on him via the monitor. He seemed to know whenever I finally fell asleep because that's when the alarm would go off. I'd have to jump out of bed and rush to his room, where I'd find him with one leg dangling over the side rail, testing to see if he could sneak out of bed before I heard him.

After weeks of sleepless nights, we finally had a good day. He was awake for almost all of it and remained calm even at sundown. I hoped to finally get a good night's sleep. It wasn't to be.

"What are you doing?" I snapped, tears of frustration forming in my eyes after the piercing alarm wakened me for the third time.

"I have to pee."

"Why didn't you call me?"

"I didn't want to bother you."

"Calling me to help you to the toilet is not a bother. Waking up to the screeching alarm every night is a bother. Come on, I'll help you up."

I had barely gotten back into bed when the alarm went off again.

"What do you need now?" I tried not to show how out of patience I was.

"I have to pee."

"You just went."

"Did I?"

"Yes. Do you have to go again?"

"That's why I called you. You said to call when I have to pee."

"You didn't call. You tried to get up by yourself."

"I didn't want to wake you up."

"I'm awake. Here, let me help you up."

Rodger was too weak to stand to pee anymore. He sat on the commode for several minutes before admitting he didn't have to go.

"Call me if you need anything," I said, once he was resettled.

Fifteen minutes later the alarm went off again. That time he tried to climb over the rail and got stuck. His left arm and leg were dangling over the side.

Unable to lift him, I woke Mike. The two of us managed to ease him into place on the bed.

"What were you trying to do?" Mike demanded.

"I have to pee. I called and nobody came."

"He didn't call. I was still awake from the last time and had gone to the bathroom myself when I heard the alarm again.

"I know," he said "You look like you're ready to fall over. Go to bed. I'll sit with him until he falls asleep."

"No, I'll do it. You have to get up and go to work in the morning."

"Go. I'll sleep in the chair if I have to."

I didn't have the strength to argue. I left the room and crawled into bed, praying I'd be able to do all of this again the next day.

Every night for weeks Mike and I took turns running to his bed throughout the night. Finally, Mike got fed up and refused to leave the room. He took his blankets and pillows and slept on the floor.

"Go to your room," Rodger told him.

"I can't. If I do, you'll try to get up by yourself and it's too dangerous. Go to sleep."

"She don't trust me. She makes you not trust me."

"She does what she has to do to take care of you. So do I. Right now we all need to go to sleep."

"Go to your room."

"No."

"I won't get up this time."

"Good. Go to sleep."

As soon as Mike was asleep, Rodger lifted his leg over the rail and set the alarm off. The next night I stayed awake in the chair beside him. By the time the weekend came, we were both so exhausted we stayed in our bed, hoping for the best.

At 3:00 a.m. I was awakened by a loud thump. I looked at the monitor screen and immediately shook Mike awake.

"What is it?" he asked, immediately alert.

"He fell," I said, already moving through the doorway.

This time, instead of trying to crawl over the side rail, or force his way past the tray table to use his shortcut, he managed to push his bed a few inches away from the wall and attempted to climb out. When he didn't fit, he climbed over the foot rail and fell hard.

"You pushed me!" he accused me. "She's trying to kill me."

Mike helped him stand. Noticing he was favoring his left ankle, he picked him up and put him in the chair. I straightened his sheets and blankets, then left the two men while I went to call the night emergency number. I reported the fall and explained I needed a doctor to come right away.

Luckily, he ended up with only a mild sprain and no internal injuries. The doctor lectured him again how dangerous and painful a broken hip would be, but no one expected him to take heed anymore than he had before. For all we knew, the voices were demanding he escape. Rather than try to convince him any longer, the doctor told us to give him a sleeping pill every night. I hated to give him another drug, but I agreed it had to be done.

We couldn't go on like this.

Chapter 34

The sedative allowed us all to sleep through the night, but a few days later it became obvious that it was no longer needed. He was slipping away, sleeping most of the day and night. When he was awake, he was too weak to get out of bed at all. He stayed in pajamas all the time. I or one of the nurses changed his adult diapers, bathed him, and changed his sheets right where he lay. When he did waken, I never knew how he'd react.

Often he was confused and agitated, trying to escape unseen demons. The venom in his eyes at those moments filled me with dread. Other times he was calm, aware that I was there and eager to talk. He repeated the stories of his life in Italy and told again of how, during the years he was in the psychiatric hospital, they let him do details. He spoke of marrying Mike's mother and how the boys became his life.

"You're my best friend. You know what's what. You take care of me like you'd take care of your father," he said one morning.

"You are my family. I love you," I answered.

"I love you too," he said.

I took his hand in mine, unable to speak what was in my heart. He had never said that to me and I was deeply touched.

Mike called his brother many times. He wanted to give him a chance to visit or at least call his father before he died. He never answered the phone or returned any of the calls. Rodger's brother answered, but he always had a reason why he couldn't come for a visit.

The social worker asked for Dan's phone number. She wanted to talk to him herself. "It's not as much for your father-in-law's benefit as it is for his. I've seen this happen too many times. I don't want Dan to regret for the rest of his life that he missed his chance to say goodbye to his father. That type of guilt is very hard to live with."

I gave her the number; she called and left several messages. He never responded.

Tears made it hard for me to see when I had to open the comfort kit and give him morphine for the first time. His breathing had become very labored and he was thrashing in his bed. I couldn't bear to see him like that. When I told Mike what I did, he became very concerned.

"I don't know if you should do that," he said. "What if someone finds out?"

"Someone like whom?" I asked. "His doctor prescribed it. It's there to help him. Who would question it?"

"I don't know. His brother, my brother. What if they do an autopsy and find out we drugged him?"

"Do you think I'm doing something wrong? I'm doing what his doctor advised me to do. I'm trying to keep him from suffering, but if you aren't with me on this, I don't know how I can go on. I can't stand this. Are you really questioning me now?"

"No," Mike insisted, running his hands through his hair in frustration. "I know you love him and are doing what you think is best. But what if someone complains? What if someone accuses us of killing him?"

"Who would do that? Who besides us cares what happens to him. Who has any idea what we do or don't do for him? We are alone in this, just as we have been from the beginning."

"I know. But it doesn't feel right. All my life I've been told drugs are bad, and now I'm giving them to my dying father."

"No, you aren't. I am. I'm the one you're accusing of drugging your father."

"Oh God, how can I make you understand?" Mike said.

"How can I make you understand? I think you need to talk to the social worker and let someone you feel you can trust explain this to you," I said before walking away in anger.

How could he accuse me of harming his father?

The following day I called and asked the social worker to come and meet with Mike. When she arrived, I went to sit with Rodger, giving them time to talk alone. Whatever Mike learned from their talk, and the pamphlets explaining the cycle of death, eased his concerns. He agreed that I should continue to use the morphine in the comfort kit, as needed.

While relieved, I was sad and angry to know he didn't trust me. How could he doubt me like that? It was hard, but I had to push those feelings aside. He was losing his father, and my job was to support them both.

"Do you want to be there when he dies?" I asked.

"I don't think I can."

"I understand. It could be too painful for you. A lot of people feel that way. For me it was important to be there when my mom passed away. I found comfort in holding her hand, with my sister and brothers around me, but don't feel you have to do it. I'll be there with him. I don't want him to die alone."

The following day was a Friday, and Mike had taken some time off to be with his father. He helped me care for him in the morning. Rodger was barely conscious when I showed Mike how to roll him in the bed so I could remove the wet sheet under him and replace it with a clean one. I had just pulled off his wet diaper when he peed, soaking the clean sheets. We had to start all over. The next time, I changed the diaper first and then we put him in clean pajamas and replaced the sheet.

He hadn't eaten or had anything to drink for several days. We knew the end was near. We placed another round of calls to the family. Rodger's brother had plans to go out of town for the weekend. He said he'd come by when he returned. I couldn't understand his decision. I hoped he wouldn't be too late. Mike's brother still didn't respond.

The next day our daughter Kelly came by with baby Ava.

"Hi, Grampy," Kelly said. "I love you."

I could almost hear the response he used to give when she said that, "I know. You love me all the time." The memory seemed to be with Kelly as well. We looked at one another, treasuring the moment, hoping he'd say the words one more time. He didn't speak but he did open his eyes.

Kelly held up the baby so he could see her.

"Ava." He smiled and reached up to touch her tiny hand—and closed his eyes again.

Mike and I sat with him all afternoon. When the day nurse arrived, there was nothing for her to do but sit by his side. Saturday was more of the same. I spent most of the day at his bedside, holding his hand and praying his passing would be an easy one. The nurse sat in the chair beside us, being very quiet not to disturb us. I had my head down, praying, when Rodger opened his eyes and spoke.

"Oh look. I see the mist." He pointed to a corner of the room high up on the ceiling, his eyes shining with love and wonder. He turned to me and said, "You go first."

I understood that he was letting me know that he trusted me to see him safely to the other side.

"I'm going to stay here with Michael for a while" I answered. "But it's okay for you to go. Don't worry about us. We'll take care of each other until our time comes."

He looked at me a moment longer, then nodded and closed his eyes again. I lowered the side of his bed and slipped in beside him while he slept.

When Mike came in to sit with us, he mentioned to the nurse that the following day would be his father's birthday. He was surprised by her response.

"Wouldn't it be wonderful if he died on his birthday?"

Seeing the shock and confusion her remark caused, she went on to explain. "What could be a more perfect gift than to see God on your birthday? I'll pray for him and for you that he passes in peace."

We stayed with him all through the night. Occasionally, he'd open his eyes and look for us; seeing us at his bedside, he'd nod slightly, seemingly reassured to know we were there. When his breathing became labored, I tried to give him some liquid morphine.

We were devastated when he began to cough, his eyes opening wide in fear as he began to choke. Mike was in agony, seeing the fear in his father's eyes. I quickly grabbed the suction device provided in the comfort kit and removed the liquid from his throat. Then called the emergency number to ask for advice. After explaining that his nurse had used the last of the morphine suppositories the day before, I was advised to rub the liquid on his gums. It worked, finally giving him some relief.

"I can't believe we did that to him. He's so scared. I can't stand seeing him suffer like this," Mike's voice was thick with tears.

"Look at him now. He's not suffering. We're doing what's best for him. Please, Mike, don't blame yourself for that choking episode. He needs us now."

Rodger was sleeping. His breathing was no longer labored and he seemed to be at peace. Hours passed and his breathing slowed, and still he hung on. Mike urged me to try and get some rest.

"Go lie down. Try to get a few minutes sleep. I'll stay with him and then you can spell me for a while."

Reluctantly, I agreed. Not wanting to go far, I went across the hall and slipped into the bed Rodger rarely used. As tired as I was, sleep refused to come. I lay there remembering when he first came to live with us. He was so intent on not being a burden and proving he could take care of himself that I let him take control of his medication. He never recovered from the terrible consequences of that last psychotic break. I prayed for forgiveness for letting him down like that.

I called on the two women who had gone before him, "Mom, Shirley, he's on his way. Please be there to welcome him when he crosses over."

After about an hour, I gave up trying to sleep. "Do you want to lie down for a while?" I asked Mike.

"I'm okay. I'll stay here for now."

Mike was on his knees beside the bed, holding his father's hand. I moved to the other side of the bed. I lowered the side rail, climbed on the bed, and put my arm around his shoulders. I felt a subtle change in the atmosphere in the room as his breathing became more and more shallow, with longer gaps between breaths.

In the early morning hours of his eighty-third birthday, Rodger Carducci passed away. As God said when he came to him in a dream, his job here was done.

The voices that tormented him for so long were finally silent; the agony of never knowing what was real or who to trust was over. He was at peace.

After a small memorial service and a Mass near our home, Mike honored his father's wishes and took him back to Pittsburgh, where he received a funeral with full military honors and was laid to rest next to Shirley. In a moment of incredible generosity and grace, Mike had the honor guard present the flag that had draped their father's casket to his brother Dan.

My heart swelled with pride when he took my hand and led me out of the church.

Chapter 35

Three months later Mike took my hand again. This time he did it to lead me off the plane that had carried us to Italy. He was keeping the promise he made to me when I asked for time to recuperate, and fulfilling a long-held wish to go to the land of his father's birth. We spent our first days in Rome. On Sunday morning we dressed in our best clothes and walked to the Basilica di Santa Maria Maggiore, one of the oldest and most beautiful cathedrals in the world, to attend Mass. Walking along the aisle to find seats in the rapidly filling church, I noticed a number of old women staring up at me.

"I feel like I'm in Lilliput. I'm a giant next to all these tiny *nonas*," I whispered to Mike, using the Italian word for "grandmother."

"All the more of you to love," Mike whispered with a smile.

We found two vacant seats, took our places, and knelt in prayer. I prayed for Rodger, my mother, and Mike's mother, and asked each of them to watch over her us, our children, and all our grandchildren.

After church we returned to our room, changed clothes, and went out to explore the city. We were enthralled by the age and beauty of the buildings and the charm of the people. For the next few days, as I had hoped, we slept and ate and wandered the sights at our own pace. I had come prepared. Before leaving home, I made a cheat sheet of Italian phrases I thought I might need, including: Where is my husband? I need a doctor. Please contact the U.S. Embassy. And, very important to me: I'd like a glass of house wine and some linguine with clam sauce, please. I used the last sentence often. The others not at all.

Gradually, the fog of too many sleepless nights and long days of tension began to lift. We ate lunch sitting at a small table under a tree, feasting on local salami and crusty bread, drinking wine, and holding hands.

Friends who had been to Italy before had told us to always drink the house wine and eat some gelato every day. After tasting both, we found it easy to follow that advice.

When we left Rome and began exploring the country, we were surprised by how spiritual the trip had become. I could feel a presence around me, even when simply walking the ancient streets and listening to life going on around me. I kept hoping for a message, something that would ease my troubled heart. Sometimes I felt it was so close I wanted to cry out, "Tell me what it is you want me to know!" I prayed each night, always ending with the words, "Show me the path you want me to take."

We were preparing to leave Italy for a side trip to Switzerland when a cousin of Mike's, who was also in Italy at the time, offered to take us to Assisi to visit the monastery of St. Francis. She told us how much she loved it there, and how she always felt closer to God when she walked the paths where St. Francis himself once walked as he meditated and communed with nature. After hearing about it, we were eager to go. Mike's cousin spoke of finding and framing feathers that had fallen from doves that circled the ancient grounds. She found comfort in having them in her home.

I was buffeted by a cold wind as soon as I stepped out of the monastery and onto the path. The slate-gray sky was almost cloudless. No doves circled above me, but still I felt an overwhelming sense of comfort. I imagined St. Francis standing where I stood, walking past the same trees I was passing. What a simple life he had lived. How blessed he was to know God on such a personal level.

I took a deep breath and stood absolutely still, trying to absorb the sights and sounds and feel of this sacred place, to take in as much of it as my heart would hold.

"Are you okay?" Mike asked, coming to stand at my side.

"More than okay," I said, brushing away my tears. "Can you feel it?"

"Yes. I never want to leave here. I've never felt such peace," Mike answered.

We were standing there holding hands when Mike's cousin

doubled back from her walk to find us.

"Come on, I want to show you something."

We followed her a few feet down the winding path to where she stopped in front of a rough-hewn stone altar. Behind it and on it were hundreds of Mass cards, handmade crosses, and photographs visitors had left behind in memory of loved ones. We were awed by the sight and the thought of the thousands of prayers that must have been said there. I wished I had thought to bring a picture of Rodger. He would have loved the miles of trails and the quiet solitude. What a perfect setting for him.

I looked again at the display around the altar and I got an idea. I searched the ground until I found two sticks of the right size then removed the band holding my ponytail. Using it to hold the sticks in place; I made a cross in honor of Rodger and set it on the altar. I smiled when I noticed a few strands of my hair woven around the band, linking us together.

"Pray for me," I whispered and stepped back.

We were preparing to leave when we noticed a rather large group of people coming our way, one of them in the robes of a priest, another carrying a chalice. Realizing they were there to say Mass, we asked if we might stay. It took a few moments to make our request understood, since the group was from Germany and no one spoke English. Once it was clear what we wanted, permission was quickly granted.

"One God," the priest said in broken English. "All are welcome."

We didn't understand a word of the service but it didn't matter; we didn't understand when the words were in Italian or Latin either. The Mass is the same in any language. We took communion with them ,and after the Mass ended, we stood before the altar one more time, prayed for our deceased parents, and said goodbye to Rodger.

Chapter 36

"Ready to go back?" Mike asked when the plane took off for home.

"I am," I leaned in for a kiss. "I'm looking forward to sleeping in our own bed. Why do you ask?"

"You've been so quiet. I thought maybe you were angry about something."

"No, I'm not angry. What would I have to be angry about?"

"I don't know. Maybe that I couldn't take a full month like you wanted."

"I told you when you explained that you could only take three weeks off that it was okay. What kind of selfish brat would I be to complain about only getting three weeks in Italy? And we can always take another trip later in the year. Maybe we can go to Ireland next time."

"It's a deal. So if that's not bothering you, what is?"

"I'm still trying to deal with everything that's happened in the last few months. I'm okay for a few days until it hits me again then I'm so sad I can't bear it."

"I know what you mean. It hits suddenly and you just hang on and try to get through it. But we will. We'll get through this together, just as we've gotten through everything else."

Hearing that I was all right and ready to go home, Mike visibly relaxed. Before long, he was asleep. I stayed awake, reliving scenes from the past. I thought about all the trips to the VA hospital with Rodger and how he insisted on paying for those awful meals in the commissary.

"It's not nice for a woman to pay when she's with a man," he told me once.

I remembered the day he asked if the people at the next table were laughing at him, and how relieved he was when I assured him they were only telling jokes. I smiled, recalling the day I sang to get him to put his seatbelt on and how he accused me of being crazy. I made a mental list of things to do when I got home. I'd gather up and tuck away the notebooks where he signed for his meals, proving I wasn't starving him. I'd donate the baby monitor to charity, but keep the food processor and try to find other ways to use it now that I didn't have to spend hours creating tasty and nutritious purees. The house would be very quiet. I wondered how I'd fill all the hours now that I didn't have to listen for every footstep from the rooms above, and rush to his side to keep him from falling. I remembered the hours of hospital visits and calling attention to symptoms the doctors missed. I got him to the hospital when he had a heart attack, and again when blood clots were forming in his arm. I fought with him when his sick mind insisted that he put himself in danger. I bathed him and changed his diapers and I loved him when he was at his most unlovable.

It was in that moment I realized that making it up as I went along was the only thing I could have done in a situation that changed moment by moment. I hadn't failed him. Because of what I did, he'd had many more good days than he would have had otherwise. Nor had Mike ever failed me. I deeply regretted the times I doubted him and gave him a hard time. He never wavered in his support of his father or me. I was blessed to have had Mike at my side through it all.

As for the future, we would welcome whatever was to come.

"Honey," Mike gently shook me awake. It had been four months since we returned from our trip. We were getting used to our empty nest again, and he was preparing for work when the phone rang.

"Brian's on the phone. He needs to talk to you. He sounds terrible."

I was instantly awake. A phone call at 3:30 in the morning always brings bad news.

"Brian, what is it? What's wrong?"

"Oh my God, I can't believe it. Everything is gone! The house is gone. The furniture is gone! Dad's on his way to the hospital.

Everything was destroyed! Bobbi, can you hear me? What am I going to do?"

"Brian, try to calm down and tell me what happened. Is my father okay?"

"There was a tornado. It hit after I left for work. Dad and Tammy were in the trailer when it came through. I can't get to them. The roads are blocked."

"Where is my father? How badly hurt is he? Is Tammy okay?"

"She's all right. She's bruised and shaken up is all. Dad is hurt but he's alive. They're trying to get him to the hospital by ambulance now, but the roads are a mess. There's no telling how long it will take."

"Is he going to die?"

"No, but his arm is badly cut and his chest is bruised. They still have to check him for internal bleeding. I'll call you when I know more. Bobbi, everything is gone. Tammy said she can't believe they survived it. I don't know what I'm going to do, but I can't take care of him anymore. Will you take him?"

I looked up at Mike standing at my side, anxiously waiting to learn why Brian had called. Already knowing what my answer would be, yet afraid to face the ordeal to come, I prayed.

Show me the path you want me take.

Epilogue

In the early morning hours, as my frail and elderly father lay sleeping, a devastating tornado had born down on him.

"I woke up to the sound of a freight train coming closer by the second. The wind picked me up and threw me across the trailer and into the wall. The next thing I knew I was sitting in the mud and everything was gone. Miraculously, sitting beside me in the wreckage was my oxygen tank, my checkbook and my rosary beads. I know the Blessed Mother, Mary was watching over me. I'm old and brittle. I should have died," my father said when I was finally able to speak with him hours after that terrifying phone call.

Dad suffered deep tissue bruising of his chest and shoulder. Cuts on his arm went all the way to the bone. He was deeply shaken.

"I can't think about moving right now, baby. I need time to heal and settle my nerves. I've never been so scared in my life, and I was in World War II."

"Take all the time you need. All that matters is that you are alive and on your way to recovery. Your room will be ready when you are. I love you," I said.

Weeks went by and his physical wounds healed. He and his stepson moved in with his stepson's fiancé while they sorted through the wreckage, filed insurance claims, and coped with the loss of so much.

Twice Dad came to stay with Mike and me. On his second visit he told me he was ready to make the move.

"I want to spend my last days on earth with you."

"That's what I want too. We have been apart too long and missed far too much time together."

As Mike and I watched an airline escort wheel him toward the security gates I knew in my heart he would not be back. He loved living in Florida and change was just too hard for him to cope with. Finally, when he called to explain again why he needed a bit more time I said, "Dad, it's okay to stay where you are. I would rather have you there missing me than sitting in my kitchen wishing you were still in Florida."

When my father passed away peacefully with his stepson at his side, I was grateful for the time he and I had been granted to reconnect. My heart no longer ached with longing for the father who walked away from me.

He had his path to walk and I had mine. God allowed them to merge and part again when the time was right.

Now that I'm no longer an active caregiver my mission is to support the millions of caregivers now doing the most difficult job they will ever love. Book two in my Caregiver series is in the planning stages. For updates on the book's progress and to read my blog, The Imperfect Caregiver, go to http://theimperfectcaregiver. com. More of my writing can be found on AgingCare.com, www. agingcare.com, and The Caregiver Space, www.thecaregiverspace.org

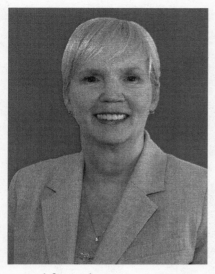

Bobbi Carducci

is a former senior staff writer for the Purcellville Gazette, a small Washington, D.C. area newspaper. Her short stories appear in the *Chicken Soup for the Soul* and *Cup of Comfort* Anthologies as well is in print and online magazines.

Bobbi's book for young readers, *Storee Wryter Gets a Dog*, received both a Mom's Choice Award for and a Living Now Award for Excellence. It was also named A Best Dog Book for Young Readers by Cesar Milan, The Dog Whisperer.

For three years she wrote a monthly book review column for About Families Publications before resigning to concentrate on writing *Confessions of an Imperfect Caregiver* and her blog, The Imperfect Caregiver (http://theimperfectcaregiver.wordpress.com/). Bobbi also writes monthly posts on caregiving for AgingCare.com and The Caregiver Space (.org).

Bobbi serves on the Board of Directors of Pennwriters, a national writers group with over 400 members, a position she has held for eleven years. In 2014 she received the Pennwriters Meritorious Service Award in recognition of her continuing support of the organization. She was the luncheon keynote speaker at the Pennwriters Annual Conference in 2013. She serves as a judge for the annual Benjamin Franklin Book Awards.

In her capacity as Founder and Executive Director of the Young Voices Foundation, a 501 (c) (3) educational nonprofit established to mentor young writers, she created the Young Voices Awards honoring books that inspire, mentor and/or educate readers of all ages.

www.youngvoicesfoundation.org and www.youngvoicesawards.com

PERSONAL INFORMATION

Bobbi Carducci lives in Round Hill, Virginia with her husband, Michael. When not writing, Bobbi enjoys the company of her family and friends, frequently inviting them to join her for a glass of wine and storytelling on the deck of her home overlooking the Blue Ridge Mountains. You may contact her directly via email at bcarducci@comcast.net.